Pediatrics at Iowa

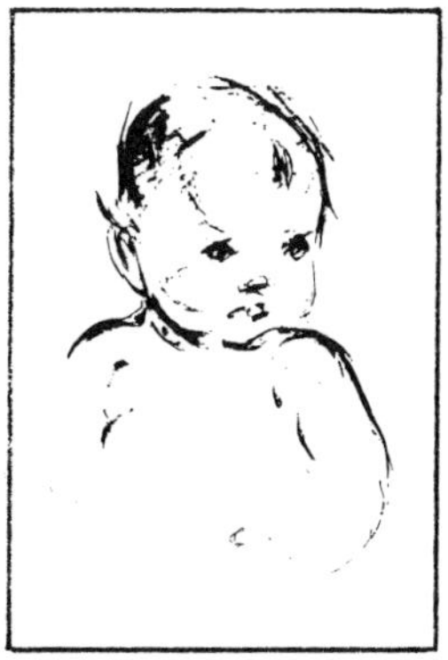

A History of the DEPARTMENT OF PEDIATRICS University of Iowa Hospitals & Clinics 1870 - 1986

PAUL B. McCRAY, Jr., M.D.

Library of Congress Cataloging-in-Publication Data

McCray, Paul B., 1954–
A history of the Department of Pediatrics,
University of Iowa Hospitals & Clinics, 1870–1986.

Bibliography: p.
1. University of Iowa. Hospitals and Clinics.
Dept. of Pediatrics—History. 2. Deans (in schools)—
Iowa—Biography. 3. Pediatricians—Iowa—Biography.
I. University of Iowa. Hospitals and Clinics. Dept.
of Pediatrics. II. Title. [DNLM: 1. Hospital
Departments—history—Iowa. 2. Pediatrics—history—
Iowa. WS 28 AI8 I6U5M]
RJ84.U6M33 1987 362.1'9892'0009777 87-10838
ISBN 0-87414-053-6

To the Memory of
Paul B. McCray and
Dr. James H. Firestone

"In the continual remembrance of a glorious past, individuals and nations find their noblest inspiration."

Sir William Osler (1849–1919)
Aequanimitas, with other Addresses, "The Leaven of Science"

"Each institution must develop along its own lines. Each one will be the result of policies which are laid down by the trustees or the board of managers and carried to their fulfillment by the organized personnel. Individual hospitals will grow and develop, the policies will change from time to time, but in the last analysis the measure of a hospital's success will depend upon the amount of efficient service which it renders. No hospital, however pretentious its building, however extravagant its equipment, can be greater than its medical staff. It should therefore be the purpose of every institution devoted to the care of sick children to develop a staff and allow it sufficient freedom and encouragement so that it may carry on its work to the realization of its highest ideals.

A children's hospital is a sanctuary consecrated to the healing of the sick and dedicated to the training of men and women in the art of medicine. Its staff should have a keen sympathy and genuine love for the work and for the human souls who occupy the sick beds."

Issac A. Abt
Children's Hospital Association of America,
1927

TABLE OF CONTENTS

PREFACE

This book grew out of my research on the Department's history in preparation for Pediatric Grand Rounds given in June, 1984. Finding myself with far more information than necessary for a one hour talk, I decided to organize a written Departmental history. The information contained in this book was compiled from numerous sources, including interviews with various persons associated with the Department over the years, the University of Iowa Archives, the Iowa State Historical Society and the few available written records, including Dr. William Keettel's *A History of the Department of Obstetrics and Gynecology,* Dr. Walter Bierring's *History of the Department of Internal Medicine, State University of Iowa, 1870–1958,* and Carl B. Cone's *History of the State University of Iowa: The College of Medicine.*

I have primarily confined myself to a discussion of the physicians involved in the Department's past. Obviously, the Department would never function without the help of nurses, clerical staff, administrators and others. Also, I have generally focused on Pediatrics alone, choosing not to discuss the valuable role other specialties such as Pediatric Surgery, Orthopedics, Obstetrics, Otolaryngology, Radiology, Neurosurgery, Thoracic and Cardiovascular Surgery, Urology and others have played in the care of children at the University of Iowa Hospitals.

Many people have provided help with encouragement, suggestions and information. A partial list of these people includes: William B. Bean, M.D.; William Bell, M.D.; Hunter Comly, M.D.; Mark Dick, M.D.; Hans Ehrenhaft, M.D.; Charlotte Fisk, M.D.; Lloyd Filer, M.D.; Mrs. Mark Floyd; Samuel Fomon, M.D.; Robert Hardin, M.D.; Al Healy, M.D.; Robert Jackson, M.D.; Joseph Kehoe, M.D.; Sarah Kull; Ronald Lauer, M.D.; John MacQueen, M.D.; JoAnn Manderscheid; Ignacis Ponseti, M.D.; Charles Read, M.D.; Robert Roberts, M.D.; Earl Rogers; Adolph Sahs, M.D.; Fred Smith, Jr., M.D.; Genevieve Stearns, Ph.D.; Lora Thomas, R.N.; Gene Tulley; Ruth Updegraff, Ph.D.; Irving Weber; and Hans Zellweger, M.D. Drs. James Hardy and James Hanson generously contributed the information on the history of University Hospital School and the Division of Medical Genetics.

I am especially thankful to Drs. Bean, Dunphy, Fomon, MacQueen, Read, and Smith for their editorial comments and to all the secretaries involved for preparing the manuscript. JoAnn Manderscheid has been a constant source of help and encouragement since the project began.

Paul B. McCray, Jr., M.D.

INTRODUCTION

The history of Pediatrics at the University of Iowa Hospitals encompasses the time period from the very beginning of the specialty to its subsequent development into the modern discipline we know today. Before discussing the Pediatric Department at Iowa it is appropriate to introduce this history by describing the state of children's health care in the 1870s, the emergence of pediatrics as a specialty and medical education in the United States around 1870.

THE STATE OF CHILDREN'S HEALTH IN 1870

At the time the College of Medicine opened in Iowa City in 1870, pediatrics had just begun to emerge as a specialty in the United States. It was a generally accepted fact among physicians of this era that the first years of a child's life were the most treacherous. In almost all cities during this period more than a third of all infants born died under the age of five years.(1) For example, in New York City in 1880, there were 288 deaths per 1000 live births.(2) Much of the mortality was related to artificial feeding with such problems as inadequate caloric content, bacterial contamination and indigestibility due to high curd tension. Many 19th-century reports indicate the mortality among artificially fed infants was as high as 80–90%. Breast feeding was clearly superior; in fact it was often a life-or-death matter.

During the period of 1800–1870 there were many epidemics in the United States. The main causes of death in children were predominantly infectious diseases such as pulmonary tuberculosis, diarrheal diseases of infancy, bacillary dysentary, typhoid fever, scarlet fever, diphtheria, and lobar pneumonia.

Basic public health was in a pitiful state, especially in the rapidly growing American cities. This poor state of public hygiene had an especially bad effect on infants and children. The germ theory of infectious disease had only just emerged in the 1870s with the work of Koch, Pasteur and Lister. Neglected public health measures such as clean water and milk, proper sewage disposal, food inspection, clean streets, attention to ventilation and public education on matters of hygiene were obviously of great importance. Refrigerators were non-existent and contaminated, diluted milk was the rule rather than the exception. A 1902 study by the New York City Health Commission found that 2,095 of 3,970 milk samples, or 52.77%, were adulterated.(3) Contamination of drinking water was widespread and living conditions were cramped and overcrowded for many in the slums of large cities. The gradual fall in infant and childhood mortality from the latter quarter of the 19th century to the first quarter of the 20th century was largely due to the efforts of physicians and public health leaders.

MEDICAL EDUCATION IN THE UNITED STATES AROUND 1870

From colonial times until the second quarter of the 19th century most physicians received their medical education by serving as apprentices to practicing physicians. The physician provided books, instruments and instruction. The average apprenticeship lasted three years and there was a yearly fee, usually $100.(4)

Medical schools run by private medical practicioners gradually began to replace apprenticeships as the accepted form of medical training in the 1830s. Very few medical colleges affiliated with universities were in existence at this time. Medical schools were largely commercial ventures, and many were opened in the midwest by physicians who were more interested in financial rewards than in medical education. There was really no "quality control" of these schools. American students who could afford it sought additional training in Europe. The American Medical Association assessed the state of medical education in America in 1848 and found it to be defective and lagging behind the great centers of Europe.

French medicine exerted a significant influence on American medicine in the first half of the 19th century, largely because many French articles were translated and published in American journals. Many American students studied in Paris. The French schools of this time initiated the era of modern medicine, developing the scientific approach to medicine, identifying diseases by symptoms as well as by lesions found at autopsy; and the importance of clinical observation was stressed. Pierre C. A. Louis (1787–1872) used medical statistics to refute conclusively the value of such time-honored but unproven therapies as bleeding, and he was first to use a watch with a second hand to time the pulse. He influenced the development of medical science in the eastern United States through the many Americans who studied with him in Paris. In 1802 the first hospital exclusively for the care of children had opened in Paris—the *"Hospital des Enfants Malades."*

During the second half of the 19th century the Germans became the principal writers on pediatrics, replacing the French who had dominated the first half-century. The Germans were largely responsible for the development of the laboratory approach to pediatrics, emphasizing physiology, chemistry, pathology, pharmacology and hygiene. German pediatricians were also the first to formulate an exact classification of the diseases of infants and determine the metabolic and caloric needs of normal and abnormal infants. This knowledge led to the development of the calorimetric method of infant feeding.

The therapeutic armamentarium available to the physician caring for children at the end of the 19th century had no antibiotics, intravenous fluids, and most of the drugs and therapies taken for granted today. The therapeutic mainstays were cathartics (calomel), emetics (tar-

tar, ipecac), blood letting, blistering and opium. C.G. Kerley, writing in 1901, stated, "I have learned that there are just four drugs that may be relied upon to serve us in summer diarrhea. These are calomel, castor oil, bismuth and opium."(5) The precarious state of children's health of the time was described well by an anonymous German author:

> Most physicians did not know at all how to deal with sick children, and many of them admitted it frankly. In fact, there were some who declared that nobody should call them to small children, especially newly borns or infants when they fall ill. Such children would not be able to tell them anything or supply them any information, and midwives and old women knew more about them than physicians. A newborn baby, an infant, should not be regarded as existing, but rather as loaned, and one should leave it to chance whether it would outlive an illness.(6)

As the 20th century began there were only a few physicians devoting themselves to the care of infants and children, and probably not more than 50 medical practitioners in the whole country took special interest in this age group.(7) Possibly one doctor out of every 2,500 in the United States could be called a pediatrician. In contrast, the American Academy of Pediatrics membership included over 29,556 physicians in 1986.

THE DEVELOPMENT AND EMERGENCE OF PEDIATRICS AS A SPECIALTY

The word pediatrician was not coined until the end of the 19th century. From about 1875 on, physicians caring for children were generally known as pediatrists, and this term persisted into the early 20th century. The specialty itself was called pediatry or pedology. The word pediatrics replaced these terms in the late 19th century, probably to avoid confusion with the term podiatry.(8)

The emergence of pediatrics as a medical specialty came from the growing realization that children were not mere miniature adults. As the fundamental physiologic and biochemical differences between children and adults were realized, the importance of pediatrics as a unique and important discipline became evident.

The discipline of pediatrics in American medical schools did not emerge until the latter years of the 19th century. Before that time, problems of infancy and childhood were dealt with by departments of medicine or obstetrics and gynecology. Eli Ives, M.D., of Yale University, lectured to an estimated 1,500 medical students on materia medica, botany, and diseases of children between 1813 and 1852. His title was Professor of Materia Medica, Botany and the Diseases of Childhood. This was the earliest American academic appointment in pediatrics.(9) Abraham Jacobi, a German physician who fled his homeland because of involvement in the revolution of 1848, is generally regarded as "the father of American Pediatrics." He arrived in New York in 1853 and in 1860 he established the first children's clinic in the New York Medical College. His academic title was Professor of Infantile Pathology and Therapeutics. One of Jacobi's contributions to pediatrics was his critical attitude towards conventional but unsound practices. It was largely because of his efforts that the Section on Diseases of Children of the American Medical Association was formed in 1880 and Jacobi was chosen as its president. The American Pediatric Society was founded in 1888 with Jacobi as its first president. In 1888, Thomas Morgan Rotch was appointed Assistant Professor of Diseases of Children at the Harvard Medical School. He was promoted to full professor of pediatrics in 1893 with a "chair" on the faculty. This was the first professorship of pediatrics in the country except for an appointment of short duration at Boston University in 1890. The first fulltime professorship of pediatrics and the first fulltime pediatric clinic were established at Johns Hopkins Hospital with John Howland as chief in 1912.

The first permanent pediatric hospital in North America was established in 1855 when Children's Hospital of Philadelphia opened. By the end of the century there were more than two dozen children's hospitals throughout the United States, and out of 119 medical schools available for study, 64, or 54%, had a "chair" of pediatrics.(10)

Dr. L. E. Holt, Sr., the second president of the American Pediatric Society, reviewed the changes in pediatrics in the 25 years between 1898 and 1923.

> Not half a dozen men practiced pediatrics exclusively as a specialty. Not a medical school in the United States had a separate department of pediatrics. When any instruction was given in this branch, it was usually as an appendage to that in obstetrics or general medicine. Laboratories for clinical, pathological or chemical investigation did not exist, excepting such as those devoted to a study of diphtheria; antitoxin having been brought out only three years before, it was not yet in general use and its value was regarded by many as a subject for further discussion.
>
> The milk station or infant consultation for the observation and supervision of healthy babies had not been organized in this country. There were no public health nurses and there was not, in the United States, a state or municipality with a special department of child hygiene or child welfare. Agitation for a better supervision of the production and distribution of milk had just begun, the commercial pasteurization of milk was hardly thought of, and the value of home pasteurization was being urged.
>
> The x-ray had been discovered just three years before 1895, its application to bone surgery had just begun, and its present use in

medical diagnosis was not dreamed of. Such things as basal metabolism were little more than a name. Lumbar puncture as a means of diagnosis was just beginning to be employed, but was not in general use."(11)

One can see that at the outset of the 20th century pediatrics was in its infancy. Its subsequent growth has been phenomenal.

MEDICAL EDUCATION AT THE UNIVERSITY OF IOWA AFTER THE MEDICAL COLLEGE OPENED IN 1870

The University of Iowa's College of Medicine opened in Iowa City on September 20, 1870. The Board of Trustees of the University had approved the proposal to establish a medical school in Iowa City on September 17, 1868. This proposal had been presented by W. F. Peck, a Davenport physician, Judge Dillon and John P. Irish, editor of an Iowa City newspaper and a member of the Iowa legislature. The medical school has subsequently enjoyed 116 years of continuous activity although it has not been a totally trouble free existence.

Before the establishment of the medical school in Iowa City there had been other means of obtaining a medical education in the state. The first medical apprenticeship in the state was that of Berryman Jennings, a school teacher who trained under Dr. Isaac Galland in 1829 near Keokuk. Galland furnished room, board and access to his medical books in exchange for Jennings's teaching the local children. Arrangements such as these were fairly common in pioneer Iowa.(12)

Two proprietary medical schools had been in operation in Iowa before the opening of the Iowa City school. The College of Physicians and Surgeons of the Upper Mississippi was located in Davenport for one year in 1849. At the time this was recognized by the University as its medical department, although no funds were provided to support it. This school moved from Davenport to Keokuk in 1850 to become the College of Physicians and Surgeons of Keokuk, and this school was recognized by the University as its medical department continuing as such from 1850 to 1870 when the department in Iowa City was formed.

When the school opened in Iowa City in 1870, the faculty consisted of eight men:

Dr. W. F. Peck of Davenport, Surgery
Dr. W. S. Robertson of Muscatine, Theory and Practice of Medicine
Dr. P. J. Farnsworth of Clinton, Materia Medica
Dr. W. D. Middleton of Davenport, Physiology and Microscopical Anatomy
Dr. J. T. H. Boucher of Iowa City, Anatomy

Dr. J. C. Shrader of Iowa City, Obstetrics and Diseases of Women and Children
Professor G. Hinrichs of Iowa City, Chemistry
Honorable John F. Dillon of Davenport, Medical Jurisprudence

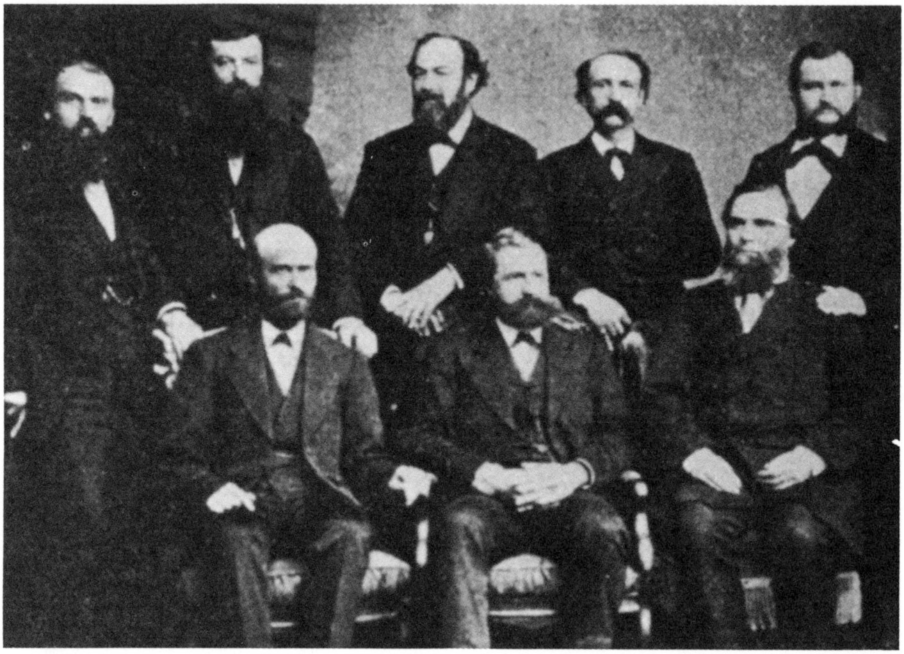

First medical faculty. *Upper row, left to right:* Hinrichs, Shrader, Robertson, Middleton, Clapp. *Lower row, left to right:* Farnsworth, Peck, Dillon.

Faculty members from outside Iowa City maintained private practices in their respective residences and came to Iowa City at specified periods to teach. They received no salary and travel expenses were paid by the physicians.

The first medical school class totaled 37 and included ten women. As such, it was the first coeducational medical school in the United States.(13) When the medical school opened in 1870, there was no hospital in Iowa City. The first lectures were held in Old South Hall but in 1873 the old Mechanics Academy was renovated for use as Iowa City's first hospital. It had 87 beds and was operated by the Sisters of Mercy from Davenport who provided board, lodging and nursing care. The need for a larger hospital was recognized but no funds were available for this purpose. In 1885 the Sisters bought a former residence at the site of today's Mercy Hospital and remodeled it at their own expense. It contained four large wards with room for 100 patients.

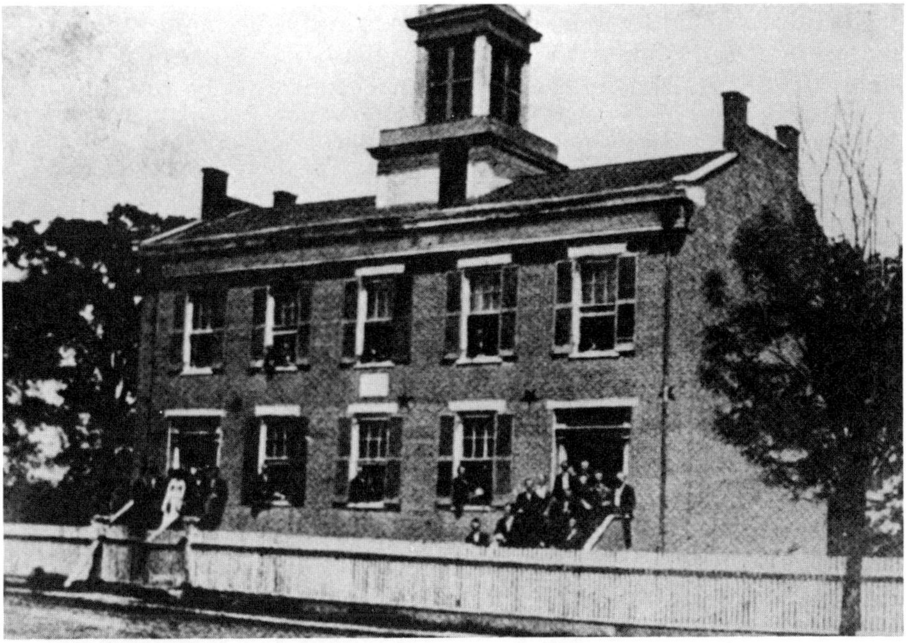

Old Mechanics Academy, Iowa City's first hospital.

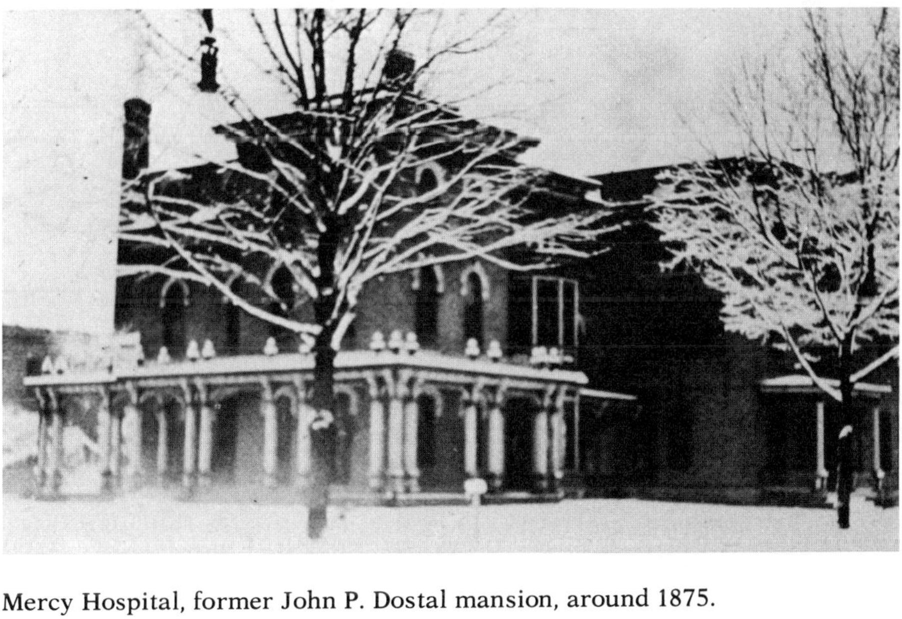

Mercy Hospital, former John P. Dostal mansion, around 1875.

The Iowa legislature appropriated funds in 1882 to build a more adequate building to house the medical school. The building was completed in 1883 and was in use until 1901 when it was destroyed by fire.

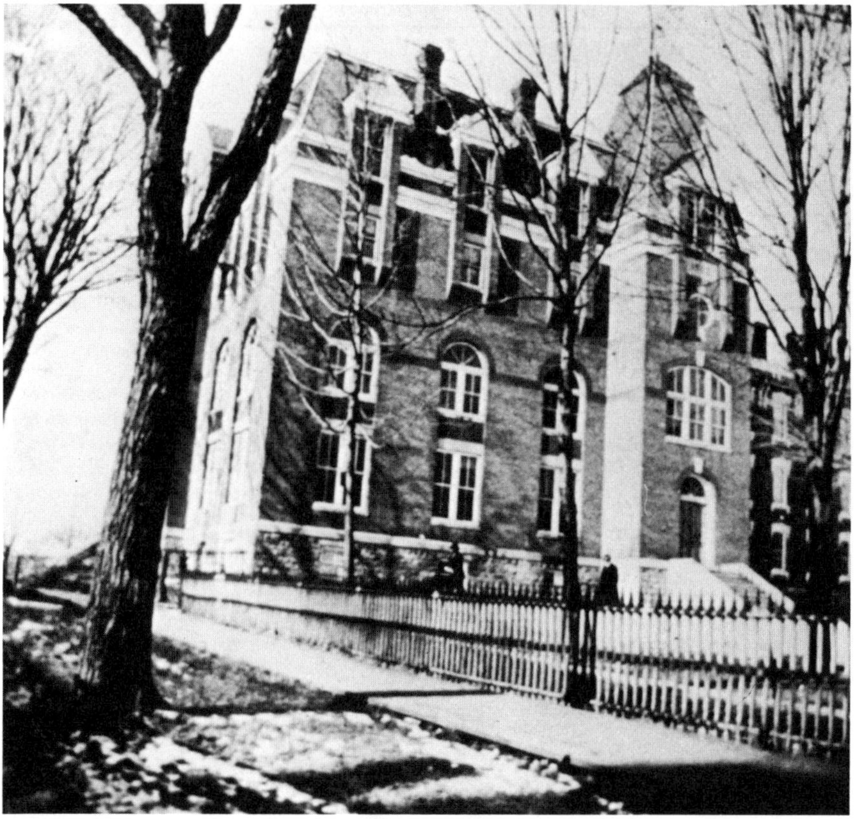

Old Medical Building, destroyed by fire in 1901.

In 1898 the first University Hospital, a 120-bed facility, was completed and opened. It was later known as East Hall and was recently renamed Seashore Hall. Three separate wings were added in 1907, 1913 and 1914 giving a total capacity of 350 beds. It provided continual service until 1928 when the new University Hospital was completed on the west campus.

On June 10th, 1897, the University's Board of Regents adopted rules to govern the operation of the new University Hospitals. Those rules concerning resident physicians, patients, and medical students are particularly interesting and are presented here.

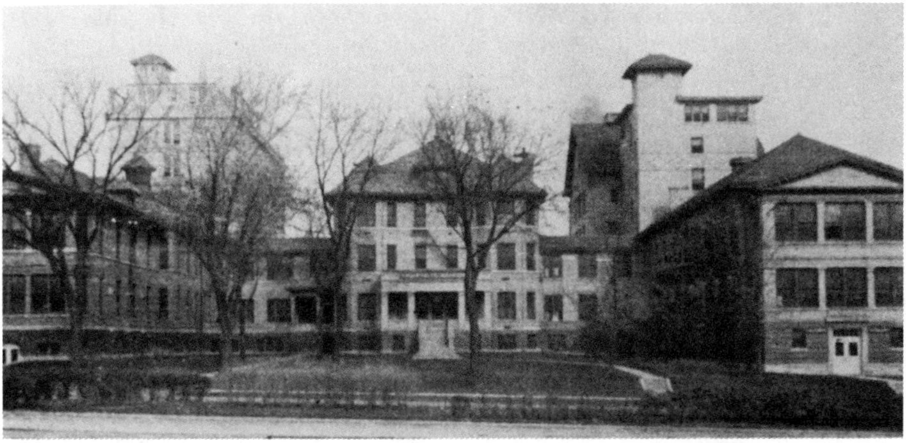

First University Hospital. (Now Seashore Hall.)

RESIDENT PHYSICIAN

The resident Physician shall, under the direction of the Staff, have immediate control of the treatment of patients. In all other matters, he shall be subordinate to the Superintendent.

He shall be a graduate of the Medical Department.

He shall reside in the Hospital and shall receive his board and washing free but shall not be allowed any other perquisites or fees. He shall not be absent from the hospital at night nor during the day except at such hours as may be authorized by the Staff. Before leaving the Hospital he shall invariably register his name and the hour of day in a book to be provided and kept by the Superintendent, and he shall again register upon his return.

He shall examine patients applying for admission and report the result to the Superintendent who shall admit them after the rules of admission have been complied with. He shall then assign them to their respective departments and shall prescribe for them temporarily on their admission and, if necessary, until seen by the physician or assistant under whose charge they will come. In all important cases, or those of emergency, he shall, as soon as possible, notify the professor or his assistant, of the department to which the case belongs.

He shall receive from the professors or their assistants all orders and directions relative to the treatment of their respective patients, and see that the same are faithfully carried out. He shall also receive from them the recommendations for the discharge of patients, and shall sign the General Records cards of such patients before they are discharged by the Superintendent.

He shall not engage in any other business than that of the Hospital, nor shall he engage in the private practice of his profession, neither shall he receive fees or gifts from inmates of the hospital.

In all cases his first duty shall be to clinical patients.

He shall take the history and keep a complete record of every case entering the Hospital and transcribe or file such record in a neat and proper manner. He shall also see that all analyses of sputum, urine, etc, as required by the clinical professors are made and properly reported to them.

The Hospital Pharmacy Department shall use all the products possible of the Pharmacy Department of the University, and the same shall be stocked up and be under the general care of the Dean of that Department or some person suggested by him to the Committees and Superintendent.

It shall be the duty of the Resident Physician to have the immediate care and custody of all drugs, medicines, instruments, and other articles belonging to the Hospital and be responsible for the same. He shall compound and make up all medicines which may be prescribed with exactness and promptitude and shall be responsible for the correct preparation of all prescriptions. He shall deliver no medicines or other articles unless the same be duly entered upon the prescription or order books, or ordered in writing.

He shall put up the medicines intended for each ward separately, and shall annex to them labels containing the names of the patients for whom they are respectively prescribed, with written or printed directions for their use. He shall deliver them promptly to the nurses of each ward to be by them administered to the patients.

He shall perform such other duties as the Staff may direct.

PATIENTS

All acute, curable, and non-contagious diseases are treated in the Hospital. Sufferers from chronic and incurable complaints may be received and retained at discretion, but will not be permanently provided for. None are received in the wards who, from the nature of the ailment, would occasion discomfort from their neighbors. Patients with contagious diseases, diseases of an offensive nature and insanity are not admitted.

Patients will be admitted and discharged between the hours of 8 A.M. and 7 P.M., Sundays excepted. Emergency cases may be admitted at any time. Patients while under treatment will not be allowed to board outside of the Hospital.

Patients must pay for room and board and attendance in advance: $7 per week shall be the ward rate except for patients sent by county authorities, for whom the rate shall be $5. In the small rooms in the wings the rate shall be $10 per week for clinical patients, and the rate in the central or administration building shall be $15 per week for clinical patients.

Private patients, in addition to the above rates, shall pay an increase of $3 in the wards, or $10 per week; and in the private rooms an increase of $5 per week over clinical patients, or $15 per week in the wings, and $20 per week in the central or administration building. The above increase in rate for for private patients of $3 and $5 does not apply during summer vacation. Patients may be assigned to the wards or to the small rooms as the gravity of their condition or the successful treatment of the case may demand irrespective of their ability to pay. The above rates are for board, lodging, and nursing. There is no charge to clinical patients for medicines, surgical dressings or operations, but a charge may be made for special nursing when required. No patient entering the Hospital shall pay less than the rate for five days. Patients requiring an operation must make satisfactory arrangements by a deposit with the Superintendent sufficient to pay the above expenses before the operation will be performed. The Hospital Committee, in connection with the Executive Committee may change or modify the above rates.

All patients who are able will be expected to go to the dining room for their meals unless otherwise ordered. Breakfast will be served at 7:30 A.M., dinner at 12:30 P.M., and tea at 5:30 P.M.

Patients will not leave their wards or rooms without permission from the nurse in charge. They are not allowed to talk to each other about their diseases. All gossiping, loud or profane talking, or any indecent behavior is strictly prohibited. Patients must not sit or lie upon the bed with their clothes on, or wear heavy boots or shoes while in the ward. No patient shall be allowed to have any book, pamphlet, newspaper, print or picture of an immoral or indecent character. Patients must not throw anything whatever on the ground below their window.

The use of tobacco is not allowed in the building except in rooms set apart for that purpose. All alcoholic liquors used by patients must be dispensed as medicine by order of the physician in charge.

Patients must be in their rooms or wards when the Resident Physician makes his visits, viz., between the hours of 8 and 10 A.M. and 6 and 8 P.M.

There is a regular diet for each day and special diet ordered by patients must be paid for extra, unless prescribed by the Superintendent or attending physician, which will only be done in cases of necessity.

Patients must upon admission invariably have a bath unless the contrary is ordered by the Resident Physician, and must have a bath at least once a week unless otherwise ordered.

The lights will be turned out at 9 P.M. and patients must retire at that hour.

A clergyman will be sent for at the request of the patient made known to the nurse in charge.

No nurse or servant of this institution is allowed to accept any gift or bequest from or in behalf of any patient except with the approbation of the Hospital Staff.

If any patient shall not conform to the foregoing regulations the Superintendent may immediately discharge him if she deems necessary, and report the case to the Director.

Private patients may be treated in the hospital by any regular practitioner, when properly vouched for by any member of the Staff, but in all cases, clinical work and clinical patients have precedence.

MEDICAL STUDENTS

All students shall enter the amphitheater by the north door.

Medical students must remember that their relations with patients in Hospital, dispensary or clinic are strictly professional, and that they must not, under any circumstances, disclose the nature of their illness or discuss with them in public or private. The student cannot learn too early that he must not "talk about his patients." A violation of this rule may entail such discipline as the Hospital Staff see fit to inflict.

If any student be guilty of any improper conduct such as smoking, whistling, singing or spitting upon the floors in the amphitheatre, halls or wards, stepping or lying upon the seats, or putting his feet on the backs of seats in the amphitheatre, sitting, standing, or putting his feet on beds or table in the wards, it shall be the duty of the Superintendent to at once forbid him such improper conduct, and if not obeyed, or when caught in similar violations of the rules, to exclude him for the day from Hospital and report the case to the Hospital Staff through the Director who may refuse the student further privileges in the hospital.

In 1909, under the auspices of the Carnegie Foundation for the Advancement of Teaching, Dr. Abraham Flexner visited the University of Iowa as part of his comprehensive appraisal of medical education in the United States and Canada. His report played a critical role in the advancement of medical education, and directly led to the closing of some medical schools.

In his report on Iowa, Flexner pointed out numerous difficulties and he made multiple recommendations. The amount of money appropriated to the College of Medicine was inadequate ($35,219/year in 1909). The College was primarily a practitioners' school with many of the faculty residing outside Iowa City and maintaining busy private practices. Equipment and initiative in the laboratory were generally good but the Departments of Pathology and Physiology were lacking in skilled assistants. A major criticism involved the small hospital and inadequate clinical material available, especially in Medicine, Obstetrics and Contagious Diseases.(14) The impact of Flexner's report was enormous and it was felt that unless the state could provide funding for proper facilities for the education of physicians, the College of Medicine should be abandoned. Several improvements grew out of this report. Funding for the College of Medicine and the University were increased. Two wings were added to the General Hospital. A modern isolation hospital was constructed in 1917. Stricter admission requirements were established for the college. Flexner recommended that a liberal and enlightened policy should be adopted in dealing with the sick of the state. This led directly to the passage of the "Perkins Law" of 1915 which provided funds for the care of indigent children at University Hospitals. Three new clinical Departments were added: Psychiatry, Pediatrics and Dietetics. The staffs of most clinical Departments were reorganized. The building of Children's Hospital and Psychopathic Hospital were also a result of this report. No single event has had a more profound and lasting effect on the quality of medical education at the University of Iowa.(15)

EARLY PEDIATRIC EDUCATORS IN THE COLLEGE OF MEDICINE

Before the establishment of the Department of Pediatrics in 1915, there were no trained pediatricians on the faculty of the College of Medicine. Pediatric topics were taught either by members of the Department of Obstetrics and Gynecology or the Department of Medicine. Only passing reference is made to these efforts in existing records.

The Board of Trustees of the University of Iowa officially sanctioned the organization of a medical department in 1848, a year after the State University of Iowa was founded. Early attempts to form a medical Department in 1848 and 1849 failed for lack of funds or a sustained interest in the idea. The original faculty was a "voluntary association of medical gentlemen" and included C. P. Hastings, M.D. as Professor of Obstetrics and Diseases of Women and Children. Existing records state that this faculty never taught.(16)

When the College of Physicians and Surgeons of the Upper Mississippi was located in Davenport from 1849–1850, it was recognized by the Board as the Medical School of the University of Iowa. Faculty included A. S. Hudson, M.D. as Professor of Obstetrics and Diseases of Women and Children.(17)

In 1850, the school moved from Davenport to Keokuk and became the College of Physicians and Surgeons of Keokuk. This was the first officially recognized faculty to actively teach as a medical department of the University. Lecturers in Obstetrics and Diseases of Women and Children included Dr. John F. Sanford, Farmington, Iowa; Dr. L. McGugin and Dr. E. R. Ford, both of Keokuk, Iowa. After the College of Medicine was established in Iowa City in 1870, the Keokuk college remained operational until 1908 when it was closed due to insufficient funds and facilities. It gave up its charter and resources and became the Drake Medical School in Des Moines.(18) Dr. John C. Shrader was one of the founding faculty of the College of Medicine at Iowa and was Professor of Obstetrics and Diseases of Women and Children. He was associated with the college from 1870 to 1906, and delivered some lectures on the diseases of childhood. An 1871 summary of College of

Medicine coursework lists twelve lectures on children's diseases under Materia Medica.(19)

Dr. Walter Bierring, Professor of Pathology and Bacteriology (1893–1903), spent several years in laboratory training with Koch and others at the Pasteur Institute. He brought national recognition to the medical school by developing the first successful production of diphtheria antitoxin in the United States outside of New York City in 1894. Interestingly, Dr. Schrader donated two of his horses to be used in antitoxin production for treating what is primarily a disease of the pediatric age group.(20)

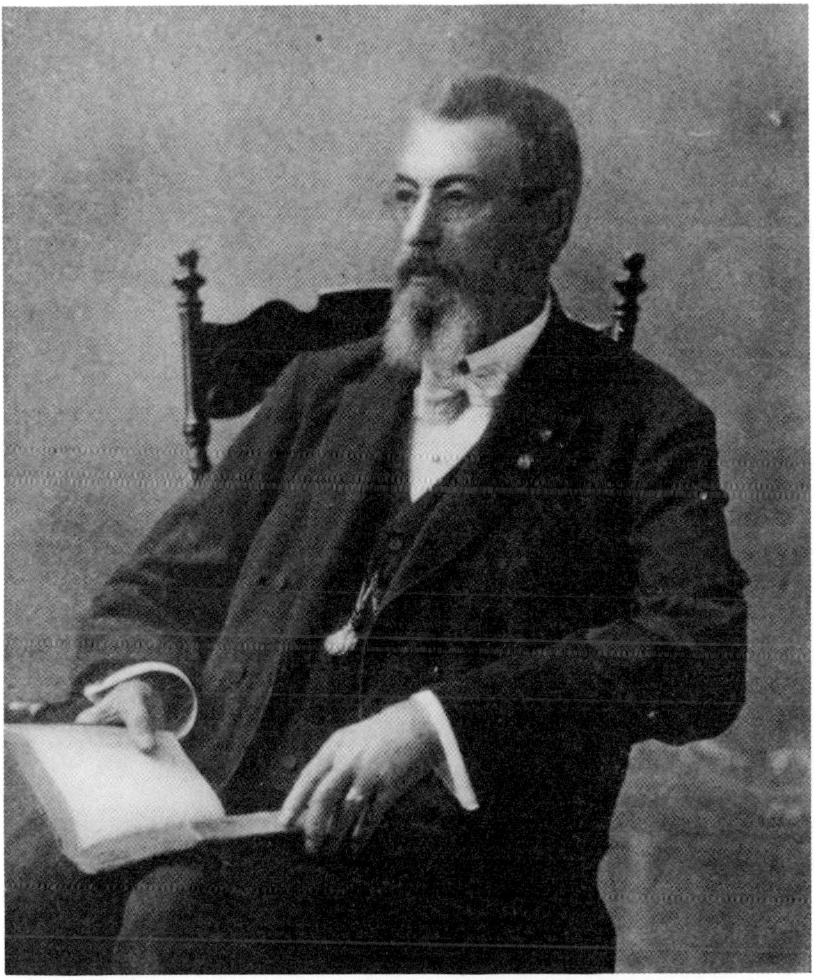

Dr. John C. Shrader, Professor of Obstetrics and Diseases of Women and Children, 1870 to 1906.

Dr. George E. Decker was a private physician from Davenport who presented a course of lectures with an occasional clinic in Pediatrics before the senior class in 1901.(21)

Dr. Charles S. Grant was a general practitioner with a private practice in Iowa City. He was born in 1872 and received his M.D. from Iowa in 1897. He had a special interest in pediatrics and was appointed Instructor in Pediatrics in 1906. He held this position until 1915 and gave lectures and clinical conferences in pediatrics. His courses were said to have been of definite educational value and he had an important part in the outpatient service.(22)

In 1915, the College of Medicine established a separate Department of Pediatrics, largely as a result of Abraham Flexner's recommendations. Dr. Albert Henry Byfield, then at Michigan, was chosen to head the new Department.

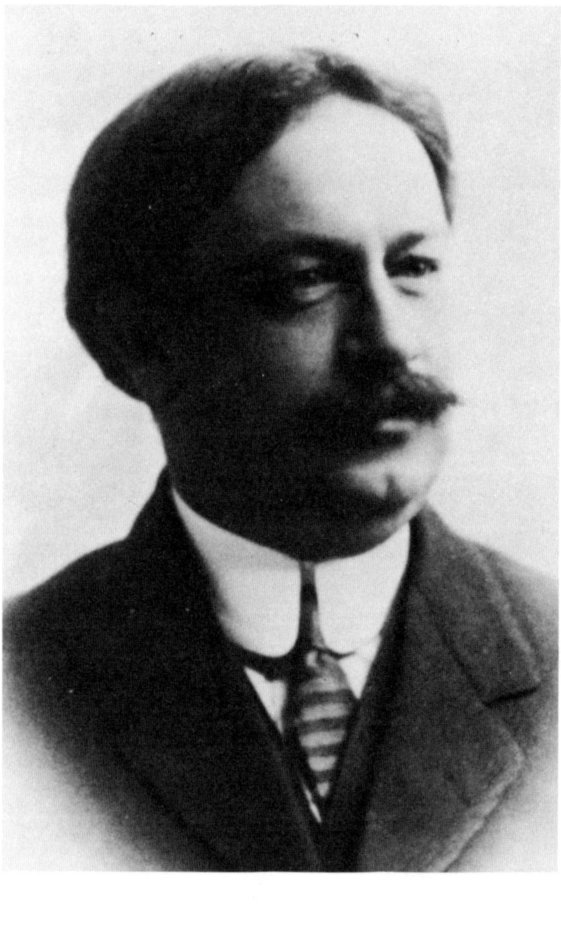

Charles S. Grant, M.D., Instructor in Pediatrics, 1906 to 1915.

References

1 Holt LE. Infant mortality ancient and modern. An historical sketch. Arch Pediatr 1913; 30:885.

2 Baker SJ. Child hygiene. New York: Harper, 1923.

3 Bettman OL. The good old days—they were terrible! New York: Random House, 1974.

4 Rothstein WG. American physicians in the 19th century. Baltimore: Johns Hopkins Press, 1972.

5 Faber HK, MacIntosh R. History of the American Pediatric Society. New York: McGraw-Hill, 1966.

6 Peiper A. Entwicklung der Kinderheilkunde. Stuttgart: Hippocrates, 1961, p. 985.

7 Smith RM. Medicine as a Science: Pediatrics. N Engl J Med 1951; 244:176.

8 Cone TE. History of American Pediatrics. Boston: Little, Brown & Co., 1979, p.70.

9 Pearson HA. Lectures on the diseases of children by Eli Ives, M.D., of Yale and New Haven: America's first academic pediatrician. Pediatrics 1986; 77:680–686.

10 Cone TE., p.99.

11 Holt LE. American pediatrics: A retrospect and a forecast. Trans Am Soc Pediat 1923; 35:9–17.

12 Bean WB. America's first coeducational medical school. J. Iowa Med Soc 1970; 60:237.

13 Ibid, p.99.

14 Flexner A. Medical education in the United States and Canada. New York: Arno Press Inc., 1972.

15 Boyd WR. A brief history of the development of the College of Medicine of the Iowa State University, 1909–1934, n.p., 1934, University of Iowa Archives.

16 Cone CB. History of the State University of Iowa: The College of Medicine, 1941, University of Iowa Archives.

17 Ibid.

18 Keettel WC. A history of the Department of Obstetrics and Gynecology, The University of Iowa 1848–1980, Iowa City: The University of Iowa, 1981, p. 3.

19 Cone CB.

20 Keettel WC., pp. 17–18.

21 Bierring W. A history of the Department of Internal Medicine, State University of Iowa College of Medicine, 1870–1958. Iowa City: State University of Iowa, 1958, p.34.

22 Ibid, p.46.

ALBERT HENRY BYFIELD
1915–1923

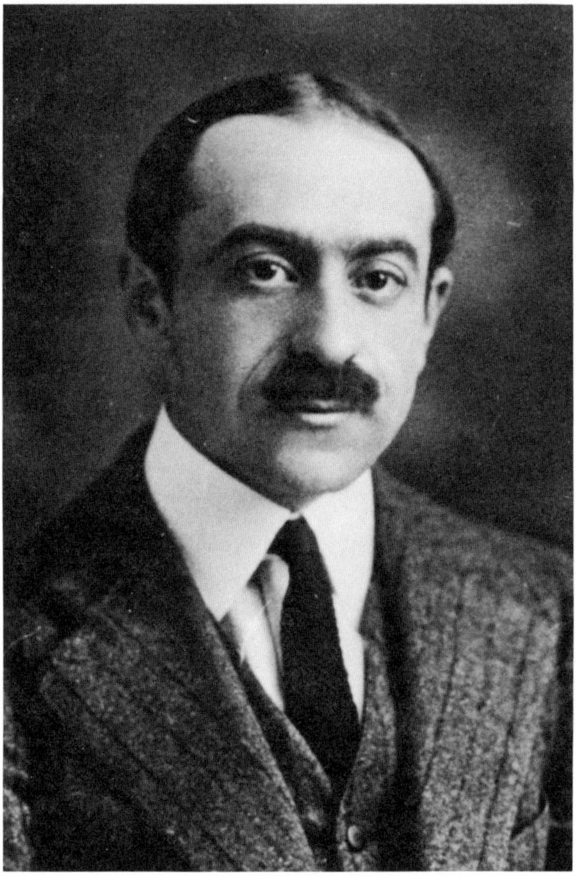

Albert Henry Byfield, M.D.

ALBERT HENRY BYFIELD

Dr. Byfield was born in Chicago, Illinois, in 1881. His father, Joseph Byfield, was a Hungarian immigrant who came to own the Hotel Sherman and the Ambassador East and West Hotels in Chicago. Byfield received an Associate degree in Philosophy from the University of Chicago in 1900 and an A.B. from Harvard in 1902. He earned his M.D. at John Hopkins in 1907. From 1907–1908, he was an intern at Michael Reese Hospital in Chicago. He then did pediatric study abroad in children's hospitals and asylums in Berlin, Munich and Vienna. In 1912, he became an Assistant in Pediatrics at Northwestern University and from 1913–1915 he was Assistant Professor of Pediatrics at the University of Michigan. When the Department of Pediatrics at Iowa was formally organized in 1915, he was chosen as the first Department Head and became the first trained pediatrician on the medical school faculty. He was a member of the Chicago Pediatric Society and the Michigan State Medical Society.

Dr. Byfield was a generous man and a good clinician and teacher. He assumed his Chairmanship of Pediatrics at a time when the Departmental resources were limited in terms of facilities and manpower, making progress difficult at times. He lived in a large house with forty acres of land on Park Road in Iowa City. He was a lover of flowers, had notable gardens, and raised goats on his land. His property included a barn to house the goats and their milk was used in formulas for some hospitalized infants. He was an accomplished violinist and played Beethoven sonatas accompanied by Dr. Arthur Steindler at the piano.(1)

Coincidentally with Dr. Byfield's coming to Iowa City, an important piece of state legislation was passed. It was particularly important for its lasting effect on Pediatrics at University Hospitals. The "Perkins Law" provided for free medical and surgical treatment at University Hospitals of children under sixteen years of age with remedial "malady or deformity" whose parents were unable to pay for their care. No funds were provided for transportation or outpatient housing. Several persons played roles in the passage of this bill, including Dr. Steindler, Dr. Bierring, State Senator Clem Kimball, State Representative H.C. Ring, W. R. Boyd and Dr. Wallace Dean. A strong force behind the passage of this law was the Flexner report of 1909. The "Perkins Law" brought a wealth of much needed clinical material to the University, resulting in crowded conditions for the patients in the hospital wards. It became apparent that more space was badly needed and this was the impetus for building Children's Hospital.

PEDIATRIC FACULTY

The Pediatric staff of this time was very small. Dr. Byfield was initially the sole pediatrician. He was later joined by Dr. Mark Floyd who became an Instuctor in Pediatrics in 1919. Dr. Floyd had received his M.D. from Iowa in 1918 and then interned under Dr. Byfield in Pediatrics before joining the faculty. These two men composed the Pediatric medical faculty throughout Dr. Byfield's chairmanship. Dr. Floyd was involved in the clinical and teaching responsibilities of the Department. He gave the first blood transfusion ever administered in the Pediatric Department. He assisted Dr. Byfield in accumulating data on an epidemic of acrodynia in 1919. During the Spanish influenza epidemic of 1918–1919, he served as an emergency physician for all departments of the University Hospital. With the aid of a local social service organization, he established a free Child Health and Baby Clinic in 1919 which was held in the council room of City Hall.

Although he was not a pediatrician, Dr. Arthur Steindler, an eminent orthopedic surgeon, was very much involved in the care of children. He joined the faculty in Surgery in 1912 as a commuter from Des Moines where he was Professor of Orthopedic Surgery at Drake Medical School. (The Medical College of Drake University graduated approximately 300 students during the 27 years it was open from 1886 to 1913. It was closed at that time due to inadequate funding.)(2) His background included extensive training in children's Orthopedics and he was actively involved in the treatment of "crippled children," most of whom were victims of poliomyelitis, spastic paralysis, tuberculous bone disease, scoliosis, or club foot. He supported the passage of the "Perkins Law" and developed outreach field clinics in Orthopedics before the State Services for Crippled Children was formally organized in 1936. He was influential in both obtaining financial support for, and the design of, Children's Hospital.(3)

In addition to the physicians mentioned, two women biochemists played important roles in the early Department of Pediatrics. Amy Daniels, Ph.D., was the first woman biochemist to graduate from Yale. She came to Iowa in 1918 to work in the newly formed Iowa Child Welfare Research Station where she was involved in studies of infant metabolism, growth and nutrition. She was on the staff of Children's Hospital until 1925.(4) While working there, she held a twice weekly clinic where parents brought children for evaluation of feeding problems or for nutritional advice. Pediatric interns gained valuable experience with the nutritional problems of childhood in these clinics.(5) Along with and independently of Dr. Byfield, she produced the first papers on infant nutrition in the Department of Pediatrics. She later left the Department to work full time at the Iowa Child Welfare Research Station. Genevieve Stearns, Ph.D. joined the staff in Pediatrics in

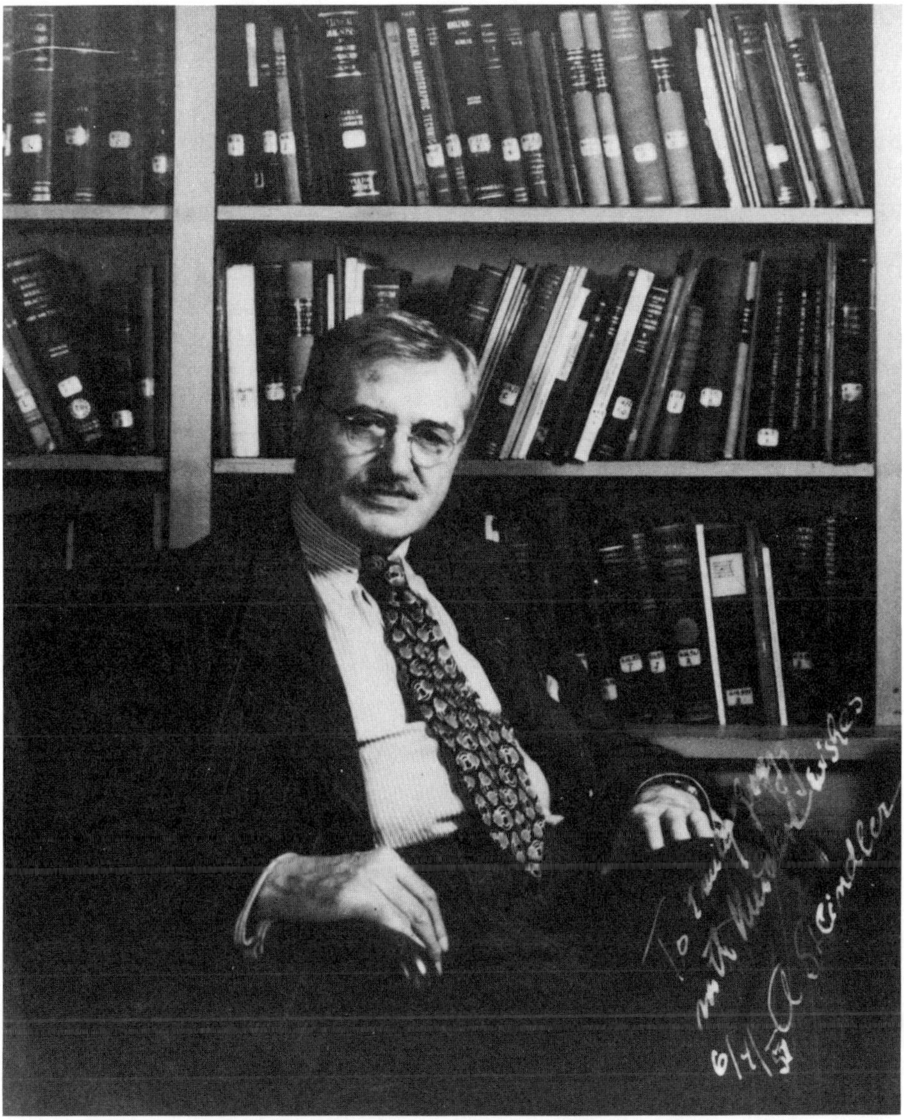

Dr. Arthur Steindler. Autographed photograph belonging to Mrs. Emily Colver. As a child, she was the first patient operated on in Children's Hospital. (*Courtesy of Mrs. Colver.*)

1920, having come to work with Dr. Daniels. After Dr. Byfield resigned, Dr. Stearns stayed on in the Department of Pediatrics and was to become closely involved in the research of Dr. P. C. Jeans.

The Iowa Child Welfare Research Station was the first institution of its kind and was a product of the infant and child welfare movement of the early 1900s. It was established with funding from the State Legislature. Early research interests concerned the physical growth of children, their nutrition, and the psychological aspects of child development. During the early years of its existence there was some collaboration with the Pediatric Department but this became less and less. The Institute received further support in 1919 with a $50,000 grant from the Women's Christian Temperance Union, and in 1928 with a grant from the Laura Spelman Rockefeller Memorial.

Among the faculty of the Iowa Child Welfare Research Station was Dr. Howard V. Meredith, an internationally acclaimed scholar in the field of physical growth, including dental growth, and one who had a profound influence on several members of the Department of Pediatrics. As will be discussed later, his data on length and weight of infants and children served as the basis for the "Iowa Growth Charts" published in 1948 by Dr. Robert L. Jackson and Dr. Jackson's research assistant, Ms. H. G. Kelly. In the late 1950s the name of the Station was changed to the Institute of Child Behavior and Development. Dr. Meredith retired from the Institute of Child Behavior and Development in 1970 but remained active for a number of years in analyzing world literature on physical size and growth.(6)

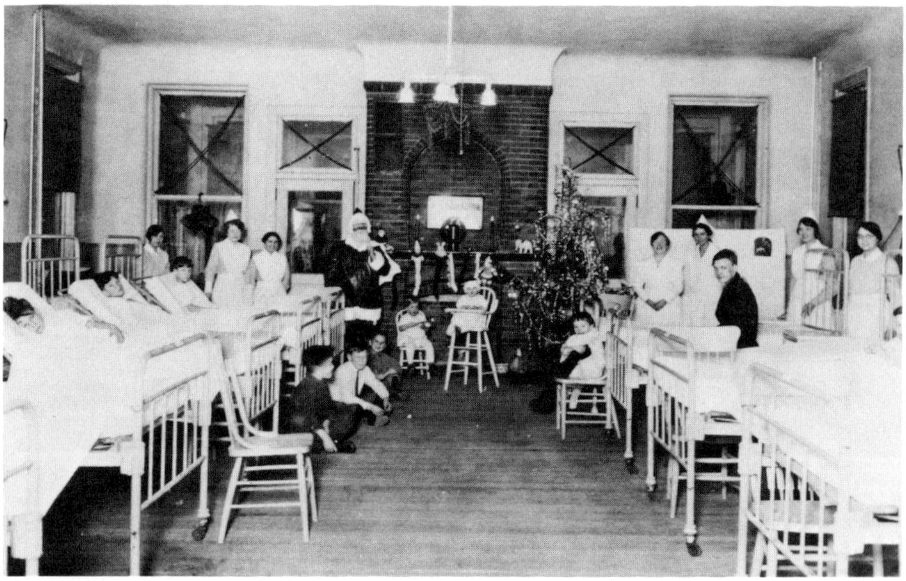

Children on Robertson Ward of old University Hospital. (*University of Iowa Archives.*)

PHYSICAL PLANT

When Dr. Byfield first came to Iowa City, the Pediatric wards were located on the east campus on the fifth and sixth floors, and in the solarium of the west wing in the old University Hospital. In addition to these wards, some pediatric patients were housed in the 45 bed isolation hospital for contagious diseases which opened in 1917 on the southwest corner of Jefferson and Gilbert Streets. On his arrival, he made recommendations regarding the care of pediatric patients and the plans for Children's Hospital. In 1915, shortly after his arrival, Byfield requested a fulltime head nurse in Pediatrics at a salary of $65 a month, as well as a dietician.

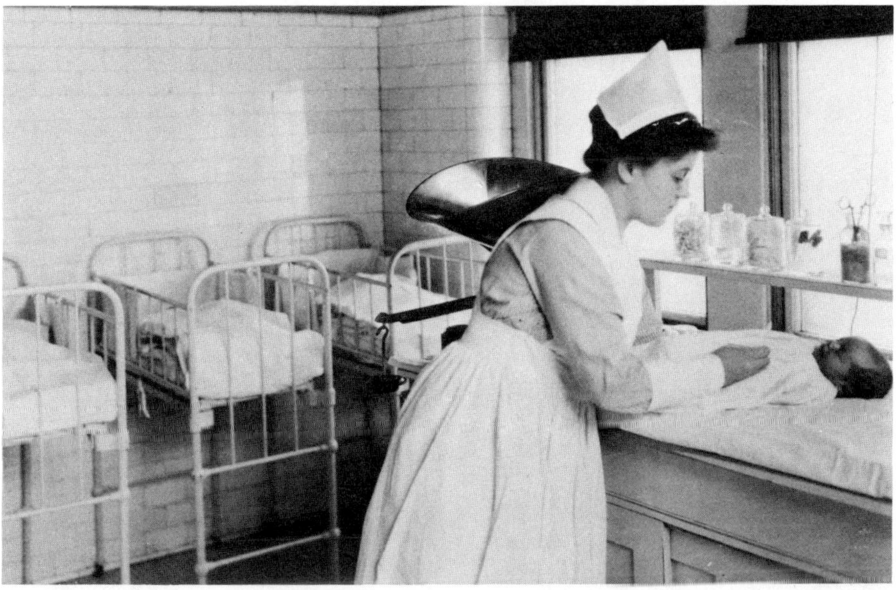

Unidentified nurse and infant on ward in old University Hospital. (*University of Iowa Archives.*)

Children's Hospital was designed and built while Byfield was Department Head. Construction was begun in 1917. It as built at a cost of $150,000 and its one story, brick, pavilion-type design was selected in part because steel was not available during of World War I. Throughout the worldwide Spanish influenza epidemic of 1918–1919, men serving in the Student Army Training Corp (SATC) lived in the unfinished Children's Hospital. Students with influenza were cared for there and the particularly ill ones were taken across campus to a temporary hospital in the Women's Gymnasium.(7) Work on Children's Hospital was completed in 1919.

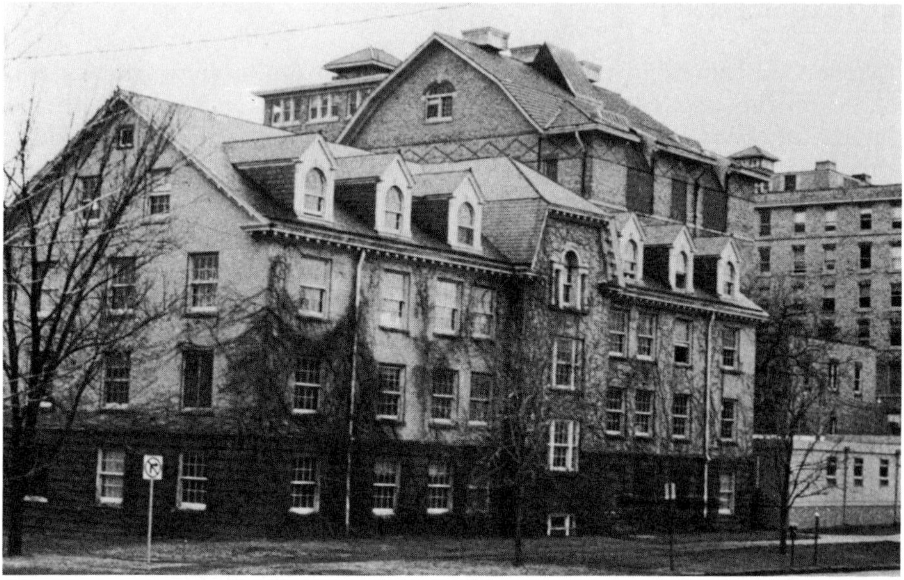

Isolation hospital for contagious diseases.

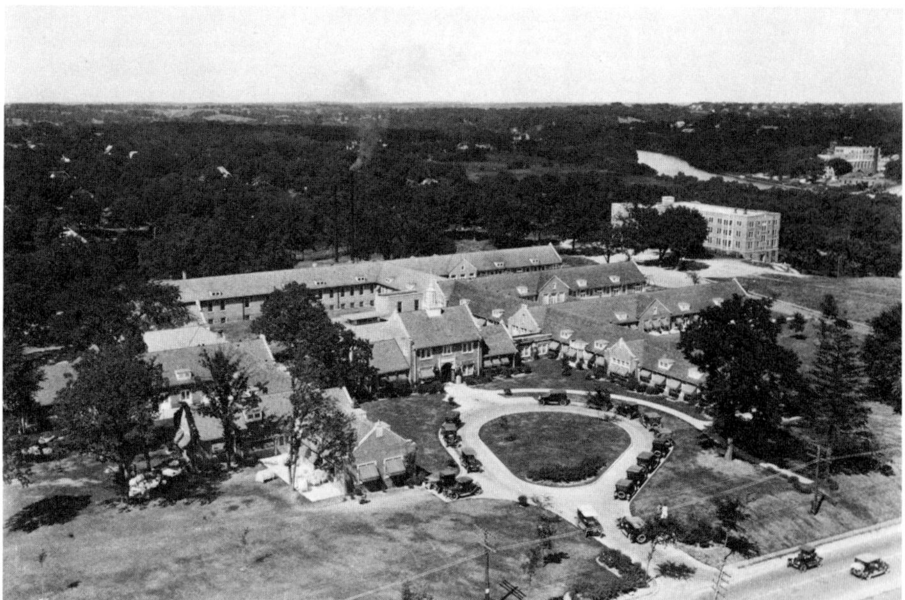

Children's Hospital, shortly after its opening in 1919. (*F. W. Kent photo.*)

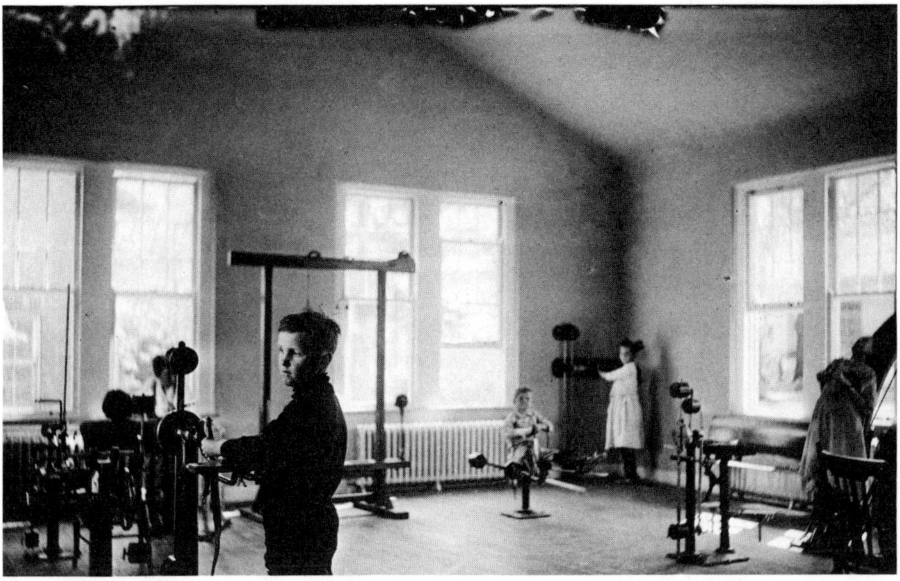

Orthopedic gymnasium, Children's Hospital. (*Iowa State Historical Society photo.*)

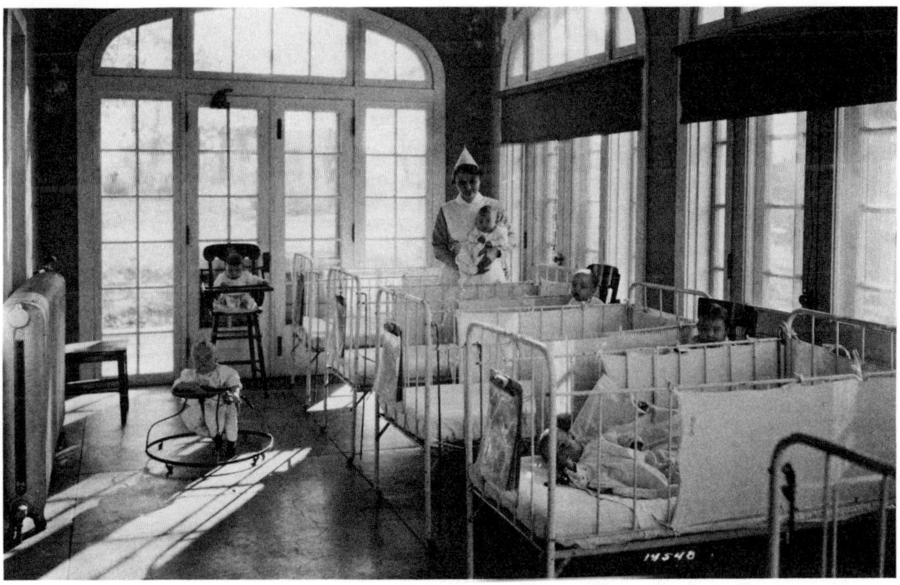

Nurse and infants in solarium of Children's Hospital. (*University of Iowa Archives.*)

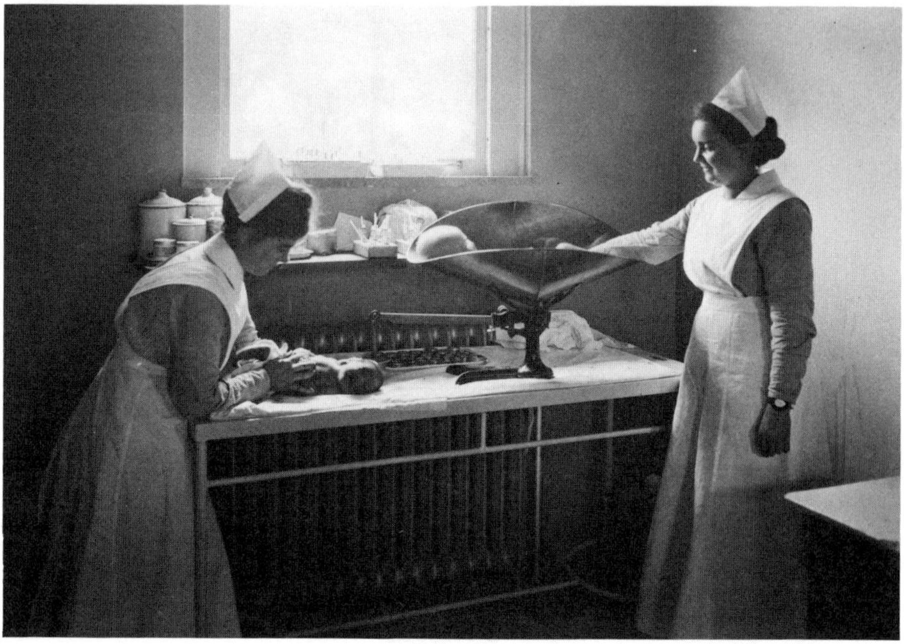

Nurses and infants, Children's Hospital. (*University of Iowa Archives.*)

The Orthopedic Department was housed in the north and south wings with about 100 beds, a gymnasium, a brace shop and operating room. Pediatrics was housed in the west wing with 45–50 beds. There was one large ward for 20 babies and children under two years of age. There were two smaller wards with cots for 12 older children and three rooms for special cases.(8) In addition, there was laboratory space and a milk kitchen where every possible modification of milk could be made to suit the individual case. The nurse in charge wore rubber gloves, a gown, and headcloth while preparing milk formulas. Sterile utensils were used and the milk was pasteurized. Some of the products of the milk kitchen included buttermilk mixture, skimmed lactic acid milk, Keller's malt soup and albumen milk, and sometimes potato flour was added to the milk.(9)

The pavilion design of Children's Hospital allowed for plenty of fresh air and sunshine for the patients and indeed "aerotherapy" was felt to be an important part of the treatment for such conditions as tuberculous pulmonary and bone diseases, rickets, skin disease and anemias of childhood. An electric ambulance was utilized to transport patients between the Children's Hospital and University Hospital.

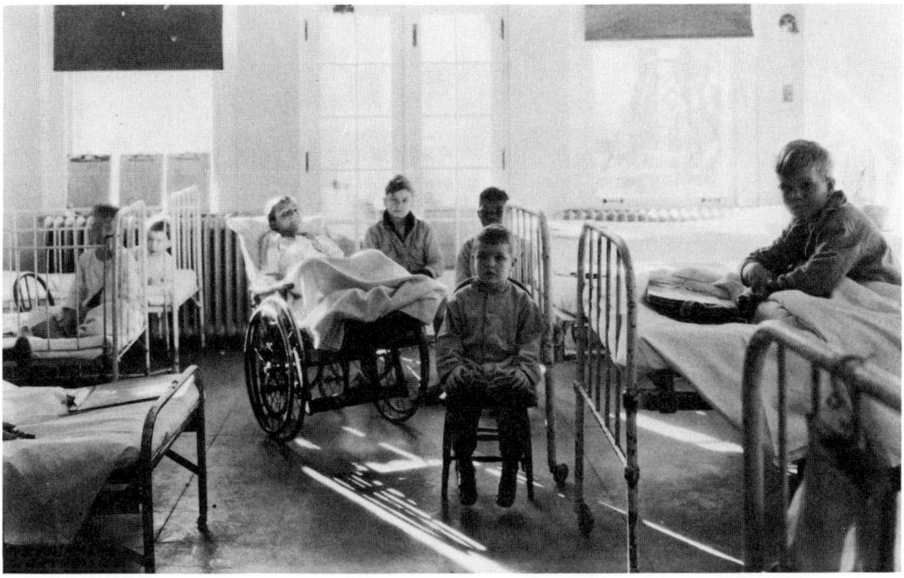

Boys' ward in Children's Hospital, 1920s. (*University of Iowa Archives.*)

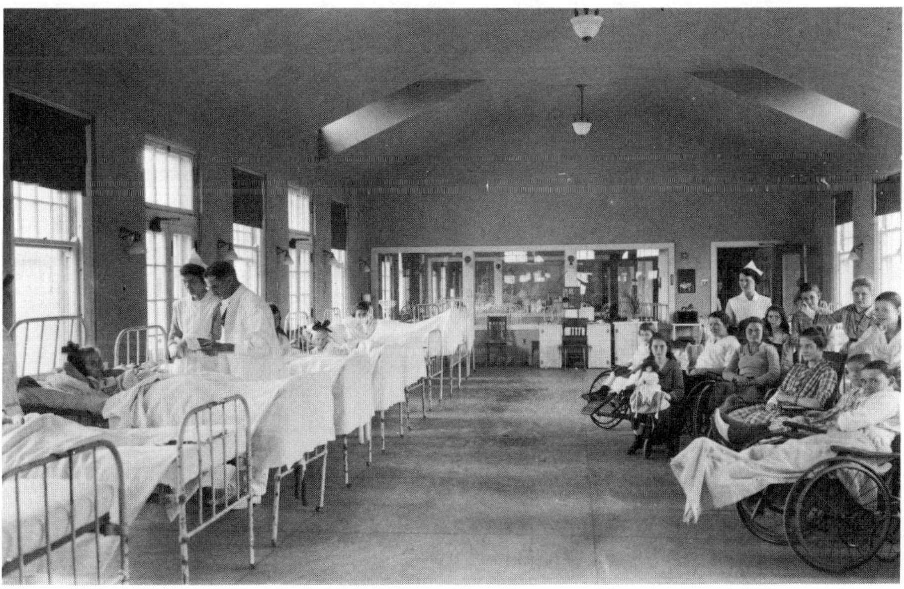

Girls' ward, Children's Hospital, 1921. (*University of Iowa Archives.*)

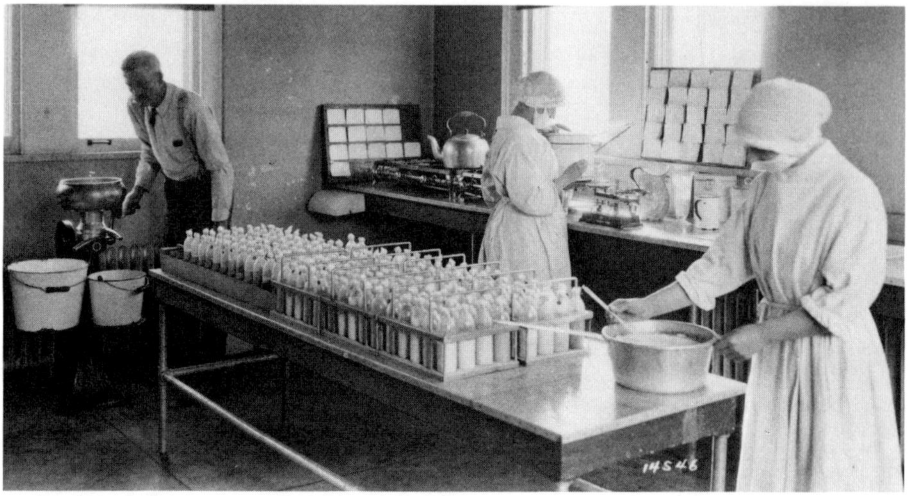

Children's Hospital milk kitchen, 1920. (*University of Iowa Archives.*)

RESIDENCY PROGRAM

The first interns in Pediatrics were trained under Dr. Byfield. According to available records, the first intern in Pediatrics was Dr. J. H. Henkin, who started his internship in 1915. Interns working in the old University Hospital on the east campus were housed in temporary quarters south of Jefferson Street, where the Van Allen Building currently stands. From 1919 on, call quarters for the interns were provided in a room above the entrance to Children's Hospital. Hospital records from this time reveal that the types of problems seen by the interns included diphtheria, measles, scarlet fever, pneumonias, pulmonary tuberculosis, meningitis, congenital syphilis, empyema, typhoid, gonorrheal vulvovaginitis, endocarditis, varicella, tuberculous meningitis, and intestinal tuberculosis. In addition, there were cases of cerebral palsy, anemia, arthritis, chronic sinusitis, chorea, brain tumors, hydrocephalus, acute and chronic renal disease, leukemia, and congenital heart disease. During the pre-antibiotic era therapy was discouraging with mortality still very high. The prescribing of various formulas to treat digestive disturbances in infants was an important task for interns.

DEPARTMENTAL RESEARCH

The small faculty of this time was burdened with heavy clinical responsibilities allowing little time for research. Dr. Byfield published several case reports on a variety of subjects including "Systemic Manifestations of Chronic Nasal Sinus Infection in Childhood," "Etiology of Arthritis Deformans in Children," "A Polyneuritic Syndrome Resembling

Pellagra—Acrodynia (?) Seen in Very Young Children," and "The Relation of Gonorrheal Proctitis in Male Infants to Hospital Epidemics of Vulvovaginitis." In addition, he published some articles with Dr. Daniels on topics related to infant nutrition. Pediatric interns were encouraged to study towards a master's degree in nutrition.(10)

LATER ACCOMPLISHMENTS

Dr. Byfield resigned in 1923, and Dr. Mark Floyd was Acting Chairman of the Department until Phillip Jeans came in 1924. The reasons for Dr. Byfield's resignation are not completely clear, but records of the Dean's Office indicate he felt discouraged about his work in Pediatrics, possibly due to limited Departmental financial and manpower resources. He returned to Chicago, where he became Vice-president of the Hotel Sherman Company and Treasurer of the Ahlbell Storage Battery Container Corporation. He later married and moved to Los Angeles, California, where he was associated with a hotel management firm called Harry Atkinson, Inc. Dr. Byfield was not actively involved in the practice of pediatrics after he left Iowa City in 1923. He died in Los Angeles, California on August 23, 1946. The restaurant "Byfield's" in the Ambassador East Hotel in Chicago is named after his family.

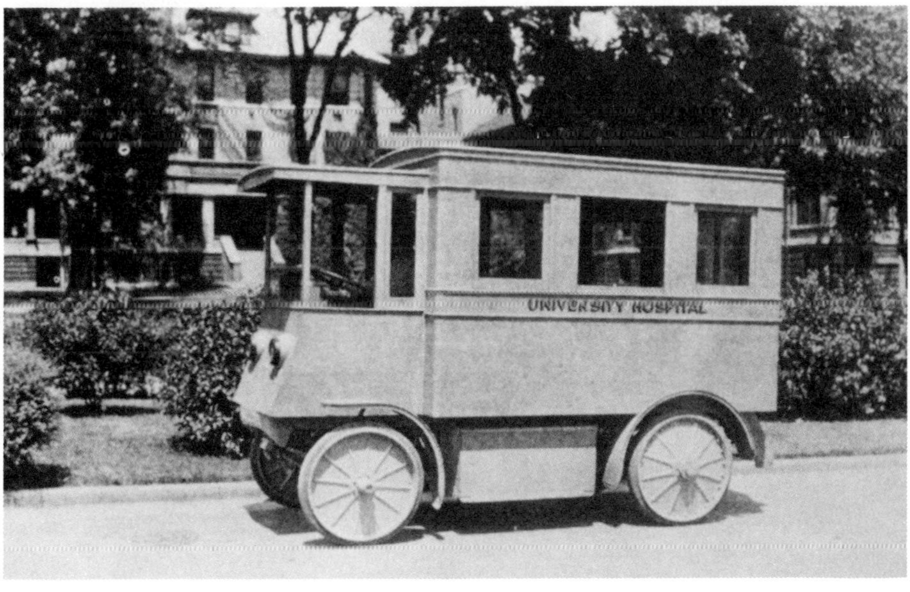

Electric ambulance used to transport patients between Children's Hospital and old University Hospital.

References

1 Personal communication: Jean Tulley and Dr. Walter Anneberg.

2 Iowa State Medical Society. One Hundred Years of Iowa Medicine. Iowa City: The Athens Press, 1950, p. 268.

3 Buckwalter JA. Arthur Steindler: Founder of Iowa Orthopedics. The Iowa Orthopedic Journal 1981; 1:5–12.

4 Bradbury DE, Stoddard GD. Pioneering in Child Welfare—The Iowa Child Welfare Research Station, 1917–1938. Iowa City: State University of Iowa, 1933 and Personal communication: Dr. Ruth Updegraff.

5 Personal communication: Dr. Walter Anneberg.

6 Personal communication: Dr. Samuel Fomon.

7 Personal communication: Irving Weber.

8 Personal communication: Dr. John MacQueen.

9 Smith GP. The Children's Hospital. The Iowa Alumnus, March, 1919, p. 161–164.

10 Personal communication: Dr. Walter Anneberg.

PHILLIP C. JEANS
1924–1952

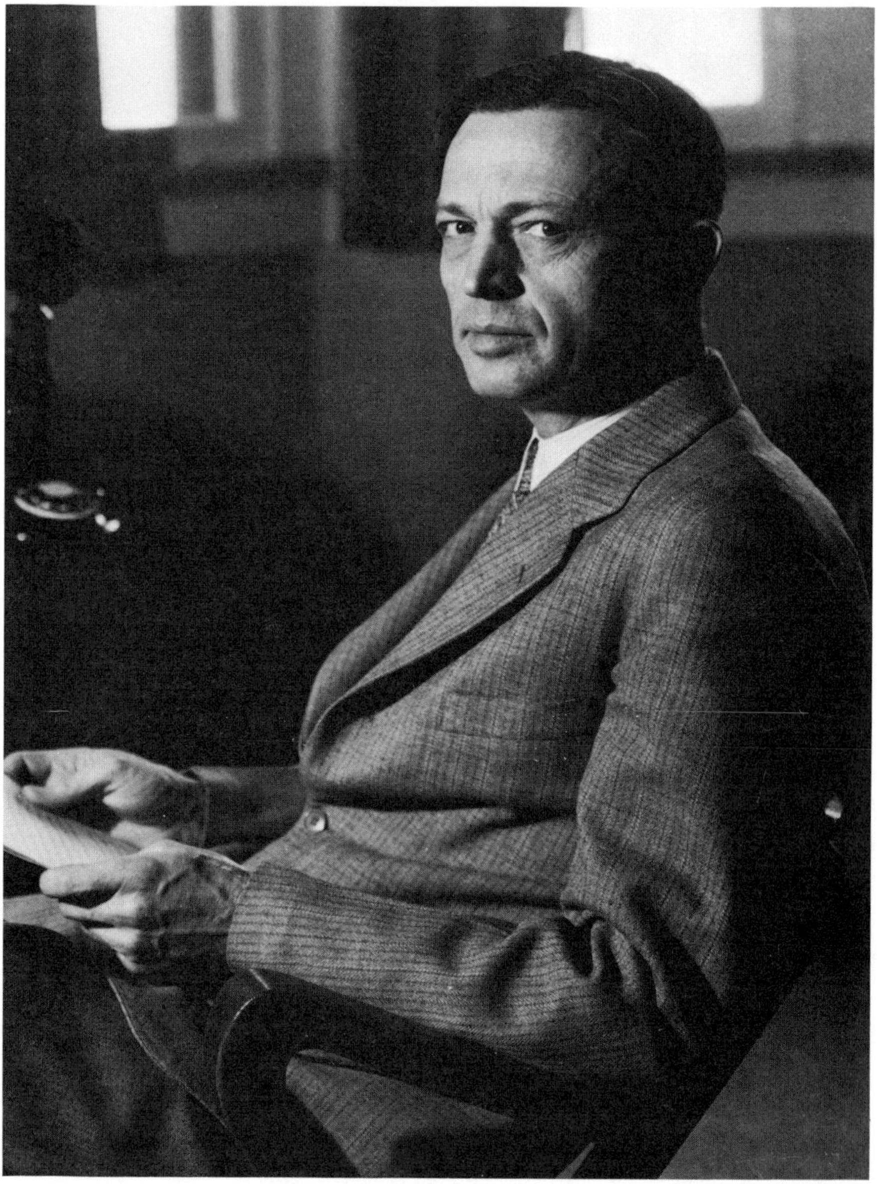

Philip C. Jeans, M.D.

PHILLIP C. JEANS

Phillip Charles Jeans was born January 3, 1883, in Hillsboro, Ohio, the son of Frank Hibben and Anna Mary Jeans. His father was a lumber merchant. He received his A.B. from the University of Kansas in 1904, majoring in chemistry. He is said to have been such an eager student that when the doors to the chemistry building were locked at 7:00 P.M., he often climbed the fire escape to continue his work in the laboratory. After graduating, he worked for a year as a chemist for a sugar plantation to earn money for his medical education. He received his M.D. from Johns Hopkins, then the leading medical school in America, in 1909.(1)

During the time Jeans studied at Johns Hopkins, two courses were offered in Pediatrics. He signed up for both, went to one session of each and quit, disgusted. His independence was obvious from early on. The summer after his senior year, he took a job at a convalescent home for children near Baltimore, where he suddenly found himself responsible for the care of many sick infants and children. He had to learn pediatrics quickly, and in the process he became vitally interested in the specialty which was to become his life's work.

His postgraduate training began with two rotating internships at Hartford Hospital in Hartford, Connecticut. The next two years were spent in Boston, his time divided between four hospitals and the study of pediatrics and other related services. He worked on an orthopedic service under Bradford and Lovett and spent time at Boston City Hospital in the laboratory of clinical pathology under Mallory. He worked for a summer at Boston Floating Hospital for Babies, which at that time was on an old ship that went to sea each morning and returned to the harbor at night to get sick infants away from the heat of Boston tenements. He also spent time at the Boston Dispensary Hospital for Children and Boston Children's Hospital. Upon completion of his training in Boston, Jeans joined the staff of the Department of Pediatrics at Washington University, St. Louis, Missouri, in 1912.

Phillip Jeans's work at Washington University was fostered by Dr. William McKim Marriott in the Howland tradition. From 1912 to 1924, he served first as an instructor and advanced to Associate Professor of Pediatrics. While at Washington University, he became widely known for his study of congenital syphilis both independently and with Drs. Jean V. Cooke and Borden S. Veedor. For years he was referred to as "Jeans, the pediatro-syphilologist." His interest in infant nutrition was also fostered by Dr. Marriott and his research in this field brought him national and international recognition. He organized and taught a course in infant and child nutrition which was one of the first in the country. Jeans traveled through southeast Europe in 1921 as Associate Field Medical Director of the American Red Cross helping to establish Child Welfare Stations. Shortly after this, his book on prepubescent syphilis was published.

Dr. Jeans came to Iowa City in 1924 as Professor and Head of Pediatrics and held the position until his retirement in 1952. He is remembered by those who worked with him as a very kind, sharp-witted, honest and gentle man with a good sense of humor. He was quiet and somewhat reserved but was always receptive to other's ideas and would listen and take advice from his residents. He was an excellent and knowledgeable teacher and was well liked by his patients. He believed in giving the residents responsibility and he encouraged research, both clinical and laboratory.(2)

In his use of language, Dr. Jeans was a precise and strict grammarian. He is said to have spoken in perfect sentences and could write copy that needed no editing. His motto was "a perfect article is one in which no word can be altered or omitted without changing the meaning." He typed his own correspondence with a small portable typewriter on his lap. His interest in precise writing and grammar led him to stimulate interest in orthoëpy (correct pronunciation of words) among his house staff and colleagues.(3) During rounds, he frequently interrupted house officers to correct their grammar. This was done in a playful manner. For instance, he insisted that polio be pronounced palio.(4) In many ways he was primarily a research person who tolerated clinical Pediatrics. He was the first full-time straight salaried clinical department head at Iowa.(5) He had no private practice interest, and was devoted to research. He firmly established Pediatrics as a research department at the University of Iowa.

Jeans wrote several books including *Essentials of Pediatrics* (First Edition 1936), *Clinical Pediatrics for Nurses* and wrote a chapter on hereditary (congenital) syphilis in Abt's *Pediatrics.* After Marriott's death he took over and rewrote *Infant Nutrition.* He was the recipient of many awards and a member of numerous societies including the American Pediatric Society (President 1950–51), Council on Foods and Nutrition of the American Medical Association (Chairman 1952), Society of Pediatric Research, Food and Nutrition Board of the National Research Council (Vice Chairman 1951) and served as a consultant on nutrition for the United States Public Health Service.

PEDIATRIC FACULTY

From Jeans's arrival in 1924 until 1937, the Pediatric faculty consisted of three men and one woman: P. C. Jeans, Mark L. Floyd, Julian D. Boyd, and Genevieve Stearns.

Dr. Floyd had joined the Department under Dr. Byfield in 1919. He was first and foremost an excellent clinician and teacher. He gave lectures on infectious diseases and poisoning to the medical students but had little interest in research. His manner was quiet and retiring, and he was very interested in well child care. He cared for the children of many faculty members and townspeople and was admired and respected by medical students and faculty alike, who sought his help with difficult patients. At Christmastime, he dressed as Santa Claus and visited with the children of the faculty. After his retirement in 1959, he continued to practice part-time and attend the Well Child Clinic until his death in 1966.

Julian D. Boyd received his M.D. from Iowa in 1921 and transferred from the Department of Internal Medicine to Pediatrics as an instructor in 1926. He was a very warm man who was closely involved in resident education and research. His research interests included carbohydrate metabolism, the management of diabetes mellitus, normal nutrition, and nutritional diseases of bone. Interestingly, he later became almost exclusively involved in dental research; and when he left the University of Iowa in 1952, he took a position to do full-time dental research in a Florida Veterans Administration Hospital. His research interest in nutrition and growth in diabetes was influential in the development of Dr. Robert Jackson's career. He was particularly interested in diagnostic algorithms and in describing the mathematical relationships of children's growth parameters. In a 1945 paper, he described the relationship between an infant's length and head circumference as 0.5 x length (cm) + 10 = OFC (cm).(6) This formula has proved an enduring and useful one. Dr. Boyd was particularly proud of a formula based on whole milk acidified with lemon juice which he used as a specific therapy for many infant problems. He was a member of the American Pediatric Society and the American Medical Association.

Dr. Genevieve Stearns, B.S., M.S., Ph.D. joined the Department in 1920 under Dr. Byfield after earning a Ph.D. in biochemistry at the University of Michigan. After Dr. Jeans became Department Head, she became his close professional associate in research and continued as such until his death in 1952. She supervised the research in the infant metabolic lab and had numerous publications related to topics on infant nutrition and metabolism both with and independent of Dr. Jeans. She recalled that the metabolic beds and boards for measuring infant's length used in their research were brought by Dr. Byfield. She conducted seminars in her home and lectured to the residents on topics related to nutrition, metabolism and protein balance.(7)

Robert L. Jackson received his M.D. from the University of Michigan in 1934 and was then rotating intern and resident in Pediatrics at Iowa from 1934–37. From 1937 to 1954, he advanced from Instructor to Professor of Pediatrics at Iowa. He was deeply involved in clinical teaching in the Department and was recognized as a good clinician and an excellent clinical scientist. His major areas of research interest included diabetes mellitus, nutrition and growth and rheumatic fever. He was influenced by Dr. Boyd's belief that the goal of treatment in diabetes should be a return to normal physiology, including normal growth and development. Dr. Jackson played a role in the establishment of norms for growth in well children and demonstrated that these could and should apply to diabetic children. He firmly believed that aglucosuria was a reasonable and attainable goal for all diabetic children and insisted that his patients work toward this end. He believed that the complications of diabetes were related to hyperglycemia and therefore was an early advocate of careful control, a view which is widely accepted today. Interestingly, the practice of mixing regular and NPH insulin later used by Dr. Charles H. Read is a modification of the system Jackson used here.(8)

Dr. Jackson and his wife generously welcomed the house staff into their home and were gracious hosts. He was also an avid poker player and frequently played with the residents.(9) He left Iowa in 1954 to become Chairman of the Department of Pediatrics at the University of Missouri in Columbia, a position he held until 1973. Since that time, he has remained active as Professor of Pediatrics. He currently resides in Shawnee Mission, Kansas, and is actively involved in the La Leche League and the nutritional problems of developing nations. He is also a member of the American Pediatric Society, the Society for Pediatric Research, the American Medical Association, the American Academy of Pediatrics, the American Diabetes Association, and the American Institute of Nutrition.

Dr. Raymond Rembolt joined the faculty in 1948, leaving a private practice in Lincoln, Nebraska. He received his B.A. and M.D. from the University of Nebraska and served two years externship at Omaha, a Pediatric internship at the University of Minnesota, and completed his Pediatric residency at the University of Iowa. The year before his arrival, the State Legislature had appropriated the funds to establish a school for the physically handicapped children of "normal intelligence" who were denied access to public schools. The movement to create such a school was largely due to the efforts of the parents of these children. This facility opened in 1948 in the basement of Westlawn and was called the Hospital School for Severely Handicapped Children. Dr. Rembolt was appointed Medical Director of the Hospital School in 1948 and was also appointed Director of State Services for Crippled

Children (SSCC) at the same time. The school initially started with 20 children who lived at the school during the school year.

Dr. Rembolt was a compassionate, gentle and empathetic physician who was also a firm administrator. He was a talented musician, playing the piano, horns, and other instruments.(10) He was an effective speaker and advocate of the disabled. His professional accomplishments were many: he was President of the American Academy of Cerebral Palsy (1960), President of Optimists International (1960–61), Fellow of the American Academy of Pediatrics, and a member of the International Cerebral Palsy Society. He died in 1983, and the Rembolt Conference Room in the Hospital School serves as a lasting reminder of his many accomplishments and his service to the disabled.

Dr. Hunter Comly joined the Pediatric faculty in 1948. He had completed his residency in Pediatrics at the University of Iowa from 1944–46 and then completed training in Child Psychiatry from 1946–47. His appointment to the faculty was half time in Pediatrics and half time in Child Psychiatry. He continued in this capacity from 1948–1956 when he left the Pediatric Department to work full time in child psychiatry. In 1945, he published the first article describing cyanosis in infants caused by nitrates in well water.(11)

Dr. John MacQueen joined the faculty as an instructor in 1949. He received his M.D. from the University of Kansas in 1943 and subsequently did his residency training at Children's Mercy Hospital in Kansas City, Missouri (1946–47), and the University of Iowa in 1949. He later completed a fellowship in neurology at the University of Iowa from 1954–56. He has served as director of Specialized Child Health Services (called State Services for Crippled Children until 1982) since 1956. He was Chairman of District VI of the American Academy of Pediatrics from 1966–1973. In 1974–75, he served as President of the American Academy of Pediatrics and was recepient of the Clifford C. Grulee Award in 1978. Recently, he was a member of an AAP Committee evaluating the future of Pediatrics in America.

PHYSICAL PLANT

From the time of its completion in 1919 and until 1954, the Pediatric wards and outpatient department were housed in Children's Hospital. In addition, after the new University Hospital opened in 1928, the 1 West Ward served as the contagious diseases isolation ward when needed. The construction of the new hospital was aided through a gift from the General Education Board of the Rockefeller Foundation. This gift was contingent upon the appropriation of an equal sum from the State of Iowa which was approved by the Fortieth General Assembly. $4,500,000 was made available beginning in 1924.(12)

Fee schedule from the new University Hospital at the time of its opening in 1928.

X-ray Service:		
Roentgenograms varying from	$3.00 to	8.00
Ventriculogram		10.00
Complete Spine		12.50
Stomach		10.00
Complete G.U.		12.50
Gastrointestinal & colon consecutive		12.50
X-ray Therapy—Complete Series:		
Long series		15.00
Superficial malignancies and minor treatments	$3.00 to	5.00
Dermatology treatments		1.00
Thyroid (each time)		5.00
Radium Therapy—Complete Series:	$3.00 to	10.00
with a graduated maximum of $45.00 for treatments beyond 5.000 mg.hrs.		
Operating Room Service— (includes anesthetic)		
Major operations with general anaesthetic		10.00
Major operations, local anaesthetic		7.50
Minor operations, general anaesthetic		5.00
Minor operations, local anaesthetic	$3.00 to	5.00
Tonsils, general or local anaesthetic		5.00
Resectoscope Fee (G.U.)		15.00
Delivery Room Service:		
Obstetrical patients		5.00
Spectacles: (approximate)	6.00 to	12.00
Diarsenal Treatments: (Leutic patients)		.50
Special Drugs: Actual cost for the more costly biologicals and vaccines.		
Barber Srvice: Per shave		.25
Orthopedic Appliances:		
Ranging in price from	$4.00 to	18.00
Body braces with head extension maximum of		45.00
Leather Torso, children		28.00
Leather Torso, adults		40.00
Plaster Cast Work: ranging in price from	.75 to	10.00
Blood Transfusion: $5.00 per each 100 cc of blood with proportionate amount for any quantity between even hundreds (minimum)		5.00
Electrocardiogram		2.50
Basal Metabolism (repeats no charge)		2.50
Physical Therapy Treatments		1.00
Sensitization Tests: (complete)		5.00
Special Nursing Service: at prevailing rates (when ordered by attending physician.)		

Children's Hospital had two clinical wards, Ward E and Ward F. Ward E was the south ward and was composed of two units. One unit was the infant ward. The most common problems in this unit were failure to thrive, congenital syphilis and acute cholera infantum or chronic diarrheas. House officers were required to write a special formula for each child in the belief that, by controlling the amount of sugar, fat, and protein in the milk, it was possible to control the G.I. symptoms. A great deal of resident time went into writing special formulas and evaluating their effectiveness.(13)

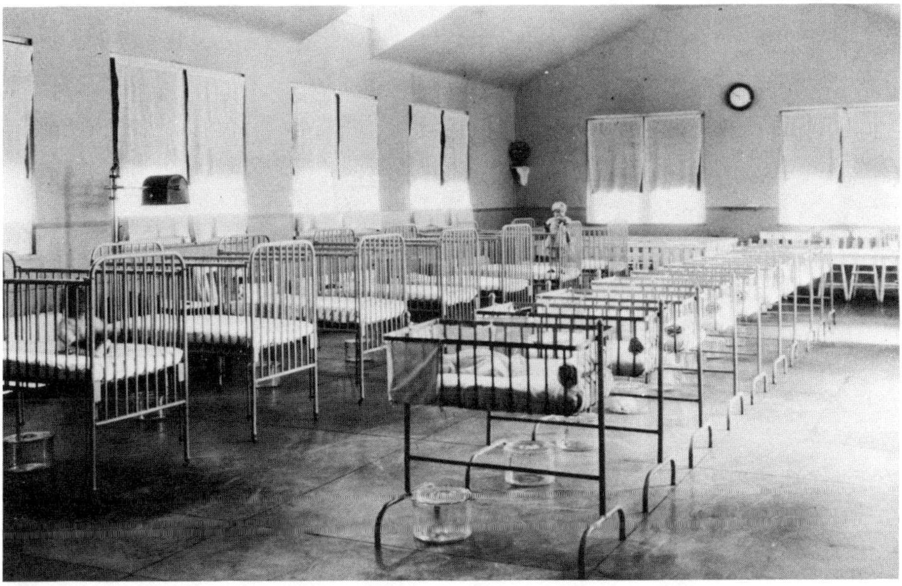

Ward E, infant ward, Children's Hospital, 1927. (*University of Iowa Archives.*)

The other unit on Ward E was an open ward of 10 to 12 beds which housed children under treatment for a variety of illnesses. Commonly cared-for problems included nephrosis, acute nephritis, acute pulmonary disease, undifferentiated congenital heart disease, seizure disorders, rickets, and what we now know to have been cystic fibrosis.

Ward F was a large open ward for older children and teenagers. Most of them had chronic diseases such as diabetes mellitus, ulcerative colitis, chronic pulmonary disease and sequelae of acute pulmonary infection (empyema, etc.), arthritis, and various forms of collagen vascular disease. There were smaller side rooms which were, in part, used for children who were very ill or terminal with diseases such as cystic fibrosis, tuberculosis, meningitis, and other illnesses. The two larger rooms were used for convalescent rheumatic carditis patients. These patients were kept at complete bed rest, often for many months, until

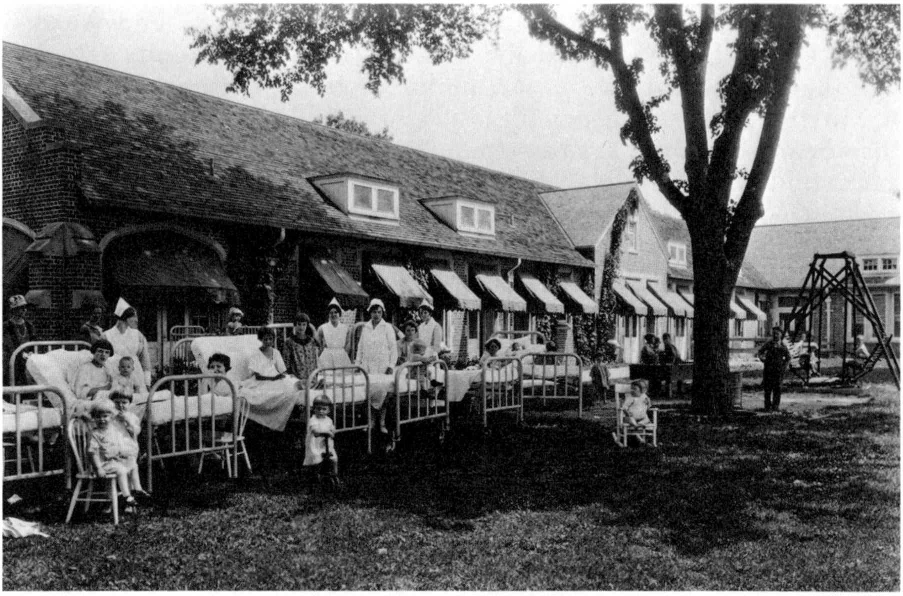

Children and staff on lawn in front of Ward F, 1926.

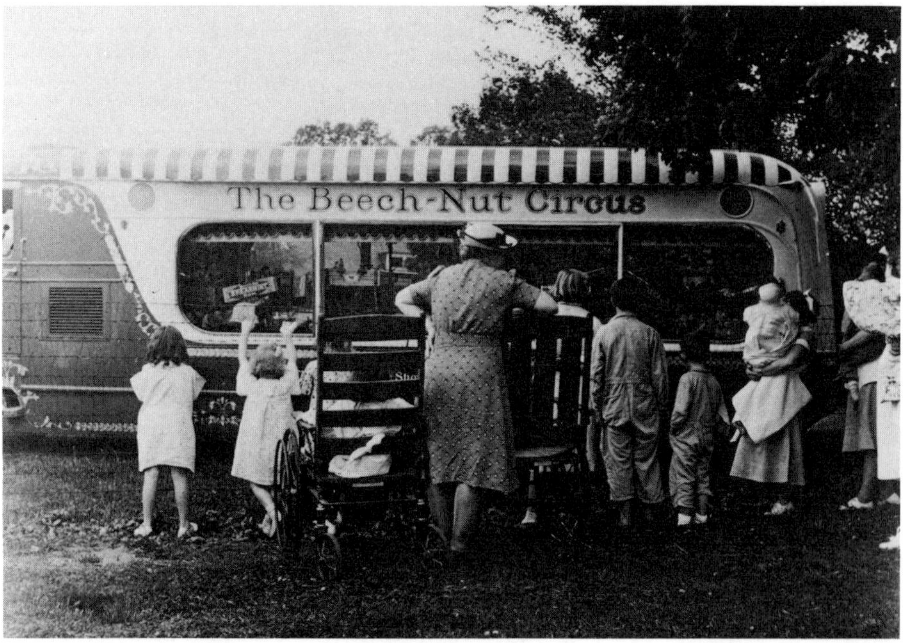

Beechnut Circus visits Children's Hospital, 1939. This was an annual event for about 20 years. (*University of Iowa Photo Service.*)

the lab work, including the sed rate, was normal and any heart murmur was "stabilized."

There was also a small area with three small examining rooms used for private well baby care. This was provided by Dr. Jackson and Dr. Floyd. In addition, there was another small area with four very small examining rooms used as an outpatient clinic. This was used to do the examinations for children to be admitted to the wards and also to provide outpatient care.

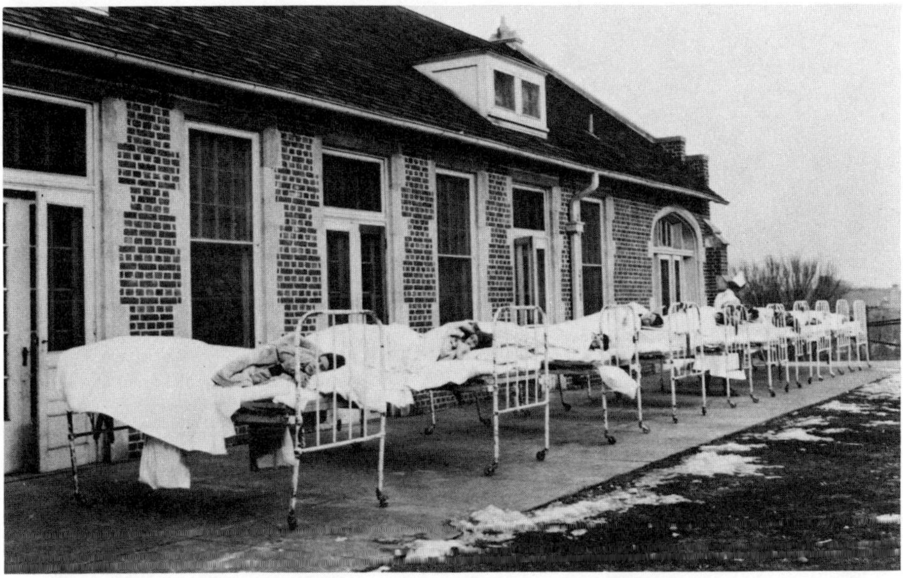

Aerotherapy was important, even in the winter months; 1923. (*University of Iowa Archives.*)

One West in the General Hospital served as the isolation ward. Patients with such problems as poliomyelitis, diphtheria, pertussis, and tuberculous meningitis were cared for there. Each summer there was a poliomyelitis epidemic. Frequently as many as 30 to 40 children with acute paralytic disease and from five to ten patients in tank respirators were on this ward. This resulted in impossibly crowded conditions and lasted for about two months. The epidemic of 1951 was particularly severe, and there were patients housed in tents on the lawns of Children's and Psychoptahic Hospitals. (14) These epidemics resulted in many children with chronic paralytic disease. Polio was by far the most common cause of physical handicaps.

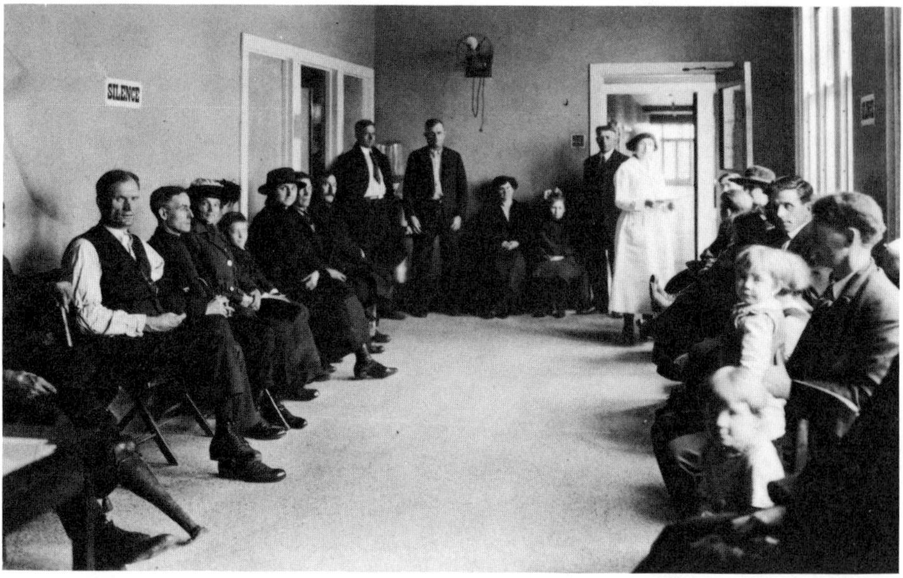

Outpatient Clinic waiting room in Children's Hospital, 1923. (*University of Iowa Archives.*)

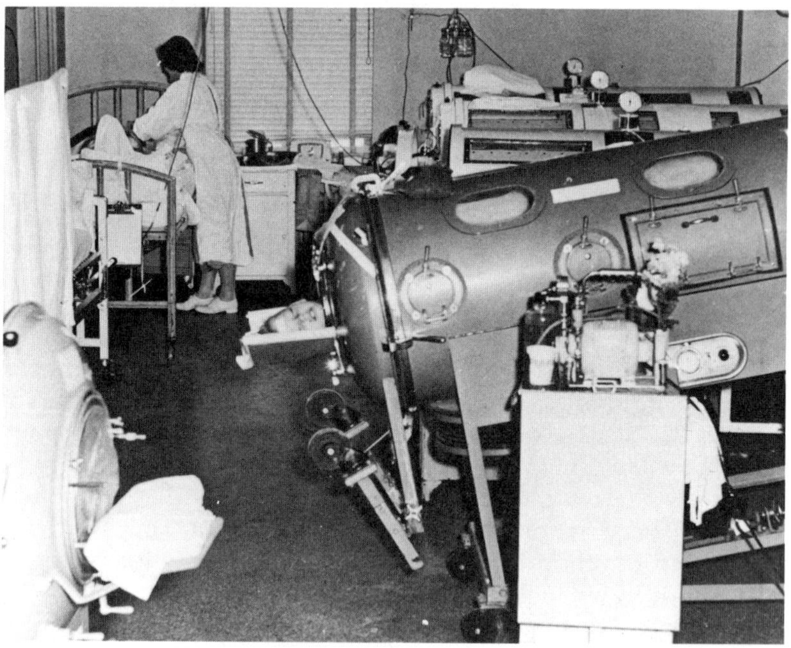

Child in negative pressure ventilator ("iron lung") in Pediatric Isolation Ward, 1952. (*University of Iowa Photo Service*)

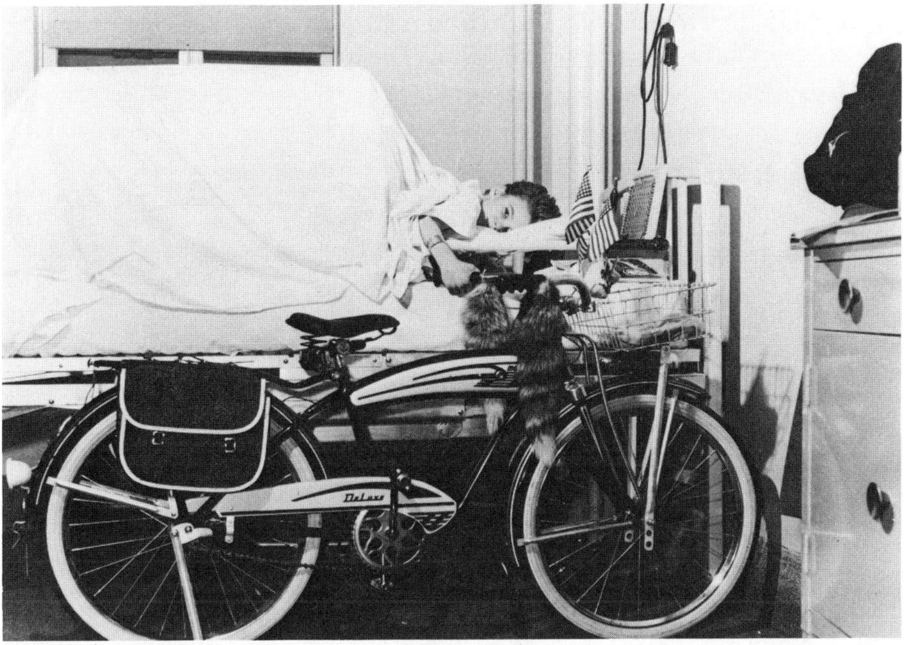

Birthday present for hospitalized boy, 1948. (*University of Iowa Photo Service.*)

RESIDENCY PROGRAM

During most of the Jeans years, the program consisted of three first-year residents, three second-year residents, and a single third-year "senior" resident. Residents were on call every night and slept in call quarters which were located above the entrance to Children's Hospital. In 1932, interns were paid $125 at the end of the year, minus breakages. Resident teaching consisted primarily of daily rounds with the staff physicians. Grand Rounds were held by bringing folding chairs into the center of the ward where all charts and patients were presented by the resident and reviewed by the staff.(15)

The interns did their own lab work including complete blood counts, urinalysis, stool examination, gram stains and blood drawing. With the many congenital luetic patients on the ward, all residents got more than ample experience in obtaining venous access to administer arsenic and bismuth compounds for treatment.

Throughout Dr. Jeans's tenure, the Departmental secretary was Florence Tulley. Her career in Pediatrics was a long one, beginning as secretary to Dr. Byfield, and successively for Drs. Jeans, May, McCrory, and Dunphy.

Erica Opitz became Dr. Robert Jackson's secretary in 1951 and later to Dr. May, Dr. McCrory, (Department Chairmen), Dr. Kugel, and Dr. Solomons (Child Development Clinic Directors). She retired after 22 years in Pediatrics.

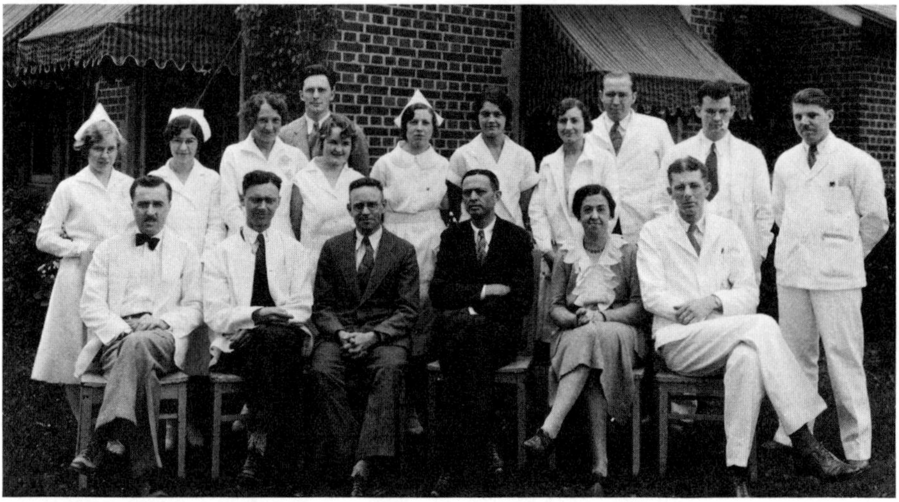

Pediatrics staff, 1930. *Seated, left to right:* G. E. Harrison, M. Floyd, J. Boyd, P. C. Jeans, G. Stearns, G. A. Paschal. *Standing, left to right:* L. Egenes, Zook, Morre, Jordan, Goff, Calvin, Catherwood, Fowler, Noble, Andrews, Allen.

DEPARTMENTAL RESEARCH

During the Jeans, era most of the research in Pediatrics was done by Jeans and Stearns in nutrition and metabolism, and by Boyd and Jackson in diabetes, growth, dental caries, and rheumatic fever.

The origin of the infant metabolic unit dates to the work of Dr. Amy Daniels and the Child Welfare Research Station which began in 1918 as discussed in the previous chapter. Dr. Stearns came in 1920 and with the assistance of Dr. Byfield, the first infant metabolism studies were done. When Dr. Jeans arrived in 1924, he and Stearns began a long series of productive studies in infant nutrition and metabolism while Daniels pursued her work independently with the Child Welfare Research Station.

The operation of the infant metabolic ward provides an example of how society has changed since the 1920s. These studies were of healthy infants, usually boys, as their urine and stool output was easier to measure. These infants came from several backgrounds. Many were children born to unwed mothers at the University Hospitals and given up for adoption. Others were from the Annie Wittenmeyer Home and Saint Vincent's Orphanage in Davenport, or Catholic Charities in Dubuque. At that time, it was customary not to adopt children until they were around six months old. Until that time, they would live in an orphanage to allow time to see that the adoptees were "normal." Babies came to the ward when they were about ten days old and usually stayed on the unit for nine to twelve months. Upon completion of the studies, the child joined the adoptive family.

Other children for these studies came from the Tuberculosis Sanatorium at Oakdale. Mothers with tuberculosis often lived there for a year or more and were separated from their children because of the risk of infection. These children came to live and "work" on the metabolic unit. Also, some children from faculty and student families were studied for shorter periods of time.

Living conditions on the unit were quite good for these children. Lora N. Thomas, R.N., began work in the unit in 1936 and remained with the unit until her retirement in 1974. She coauthored a number of infant nutrition studies and continued to work as a consultant to the Division of Nutrition until the mid 1980s. In 1974 the metabolic unit was officially named the Lora N. Thomas Metabolic Unit in her honor. She remembers that the children were pampered and loved by their caretakers. They got a lot of attention from the staff on the ward and employees from General Hospital used to come to play with the children. During the studies, the babies would stay on the metabolic beds from three to five days at a time. There have been no long term followup studies of these infants looking at their subsequent psychological and emotional development.

The studies done in the metabolic unit resulted in numerous publications. Jeans's and Stearns's metabolic balance studies were pioneering. They highlighted and promoted sustained interest in nutrition in infants. They first studied normal infants and later older children and adolescents. In the study of healthy children, they helped establish norms to serve as comparisons with the sick child. Perhaps their most important studies were those involving nitrogen, calcium, and phosphorus balance. They also studied the role of vitamin D in growth, attempting to find what the normal daily requirements were. When manufacturers began to add vitamin D to milk in the early 1940s, Jeans's recommendation of adding 400 I.U./quart was followed. This helped in decreasing the incidence of rickets. Jeans's edition of Marriott's *Infant Nutrition* was a standard text on this subject. Dr. Jeans was a national and international authority in the field of pediatric nutrition, and his work was the basis for future hypotheses and studies in nutrition.(16)

After Dr. Jeans's retirement in 1952, Dr. Charles D. May became the Department Head, and he continued the operation of the metabolic unit. In 1954, he recruited Dr. Samuel Fomon, who continued to develop and be involved with the metabolic unit and research in nutrition after his arrival here. Dr. Stearns left the Department after Dr. Jeans's death and continued her research in the Department of Orthopedics.

Dr. Julian Boyd was engaged in several areas of research, one being diabetes mellitus. It was his long-held belief that the goal of treatment should be to return to normal physiology, including normal growth and development. This view influenced the thinking of Dr. Robert Jackson. Together and independently, they studied the effects of various types of insulin, programs of insulin administration, and diets on diabetic children's growth and development. They advocated tight control of the young diabetic as a way to prevent vascular complications. Dr. Boyd became very interested in tooth development and the etiology and prevention of dental caries. When he left the Department in 1952, he devoted his time exclusively to dental research.

Dr. Jackson was especially interested in the study of growth in children. In 1945, he and Helen Kelly published an article titled "Growth Charts for Use in Pediatric Practice" in the *Journal of Pediatrics.*(17) The so-called "Iowa Growth Charts" were constructed from data gathered by Dr. Howard Meredith, Ph.D., and colleagues at the Iowa Child Welfare Research Station in their studies of 1,500 boys and 1,500 girls, most of whom were from upper-middle-class families. Dr. Meredith collaborated with Dr. Harold C. Stuart of Harvard University in preparation of the Harvard-Iowa tables of length and weight of children. The data were collected from 1920 to 1940, and these charts were widely used until the National Center for Health Statistics data were published in 1972.

The Jeans era also saw the growth and development of the State Services for Crippled Children (SSCC) Clinics. This program derived largely from the Federal Social Security Act of 1935 and the funds it alloted for the care of crippled children. Iowa's clinics were formally organized in 1936 to include orthopedics and pediatrics with the addition of a social worker in 1939, child psychology in 1943, a dietary consultant in 1948, and a dental technician and a speech and hearing consultant in 1949. Initially, field clinics were held every few years in each of the eleven districts. The purpose of these diagnostic clinics was to provide consultation and advice to the family physicians and additionally to serve as teaching clinics for physicians in training. In 1941, certain medical societies in the state requested that continuous clinics be held by the SSCC in their communities. These more frequent field clinics allowed much better followup and continuity of care for the child and family.(18)

Following the organization of SSCC in 1936, Dr. E. N. MacEwen, Dean of the College of Medicine, served as the Executive Director of the program until his death in 1947. Dr. Rembolt became Assistant Director in 1948 and later became Executive Director of the program. Dr. Rembolt was succeeded in 1956 by Dr. John C. MacQueen, who is the current director of the program now called Child Health Specialty Clinics (CHSC). Over the years, these clinics have grown to provide pediatric consultation in general pediatrics, cardiology, diabetes, cystic fibrosis, genetic conditions, psychology, speech and hearing, development disabilities, physical therapy, and high-risk infant followup.

LATER ACCOMPLISHMENTS

Dr. Jeans retired as Chairman of the Department in 1952 and became Professor Emeritus in Pediatrics. At the time he retired, his health was failing. He died that same year of a coronary thrombosis while in Panama on a World Health Organization project studying nutrition in the Central American republics. Dr. Jeans was buried in Oakland Cemetery in Iowa City near the grave of Dr. Arthur Steindler. Dr. Charles D. May succeeded him as the third Head of the Department of Pediatrics.

References

1 Anonymous. Biography of P.C. Jeans. Pediatric Library, University of Iowa.

2 Personal communication: Dr. John MacQueen and Dr. Joseph Kehoe.

3 Cooke JV. Medical orthoëpy. Washington University Medical Alum Quarterly 1943; 6:89–91.

4 Personal communication: Dr. John MacQueen.

5 Personal communication: Dr. Robert Hardin.

6 Boyd JR. Clinical appraisal of infant's head size. Am J Dis Child 1945; 69:71–82.

7 Personal communication: Dr. Genevieve Stearns.

8 Personal communication: Dr. Robert Hardin.

9 Personal communication: Dr. John MacQueen.

10 Personal communication: Dr. Alfred Healy.

11 Comly HH. Cyanosis in infants caused by nitrates in well water. JAMA 1945; 129:112–16.

12 Bierring W. A history of the Department of Internal Medicine, State University of Iowa College of Medicine, 1870–1958. Iowa City: State University of Iowa, 1958.

13 Personal communication: Dr. John MacQueen.

14 Personal communication: Dr. William B. Bean.

15 Personal communication: Dr. John MacQueen and Dr. Charlotte Fisk.

16 Personal communication: Dr. Samuel Fomon.

17 Jackson RL, Kelly HG. Growth charts for use in pediatric practice. J Ped 1945; 27:215–229.

18 Schweitzer CR. A developmental history of the State Services for Crippled Children's Program in Iowa. MA thesis, University of Iowa, 1951.

CHARLES D. MAY
1952–1957

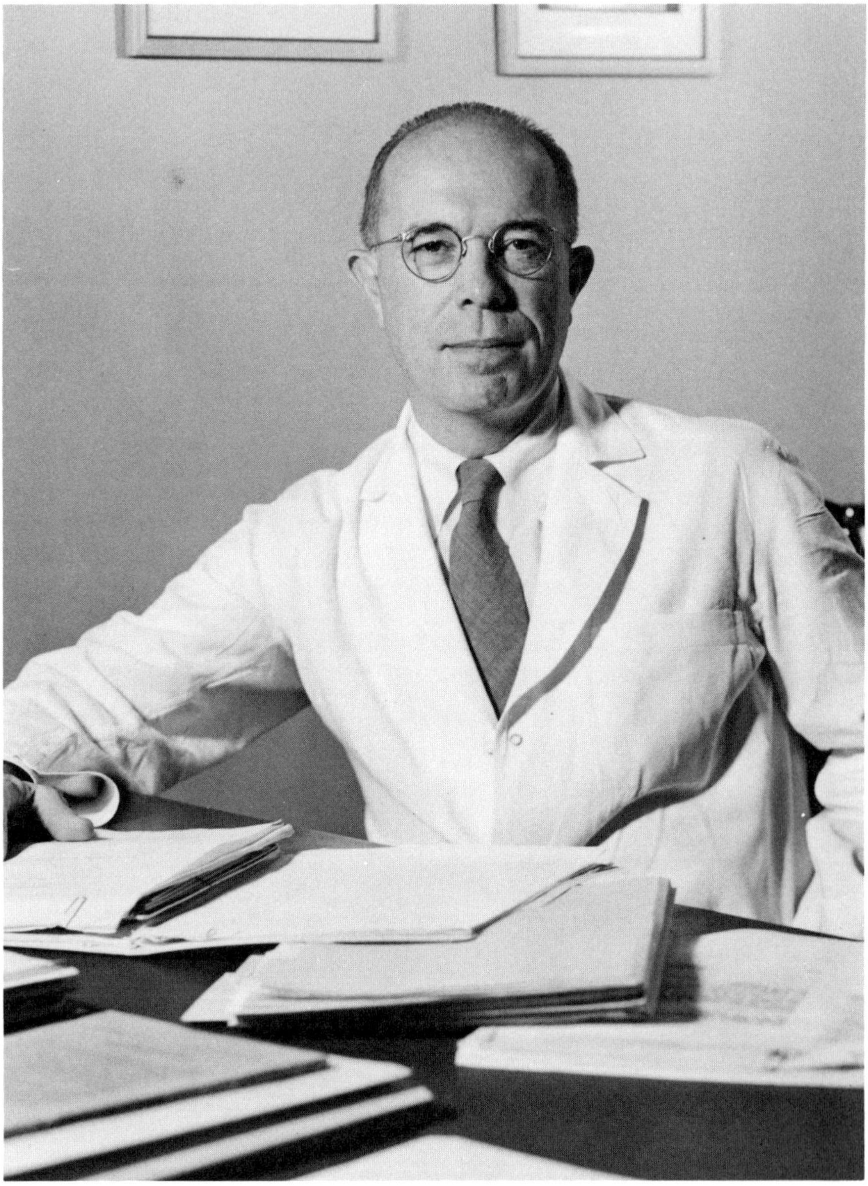

Charles D. May, M.D.

CHARLES D. MAY

Dr. May was born in St. Louis, Missouri, in 1908. He received his B.A. from the University of Minnesota and his M.D. from Harvard in 1935. His postgraduate work was at Children's Hospital of Boston, where he was a house officer in bacteriology and pathology from 1935–36 and in pediatrics from 1936–37. He was successively assistant resident and resident in pediatrics from 1937–41. In 1941, he was a Commonwealth Fund Fellow with Professor Fieser at Harvard. He served in the Army Medical Corp from 1942–46. He was certified by the American Board of Pediatrics in 1941. He returned to the University of Minnesota, where he was an Associate Professor of Pediatrics under Dr. McQuarrie until he came to Iowa City.

Dr. May's research interests included nutritional disorders of childhood such as celiac disease and cystic fibrosis and the role of vitamins A, B_6, B_{12}, and folic acid in health and disease. While at Children's Hospital of Boston, he worked with Dr. Kenneth Blackfan describing the differences in pathology between cystic fibrosis and celiac disease. In 1938 they published a paper in the *Journal of Pediatrics,* describing some of the clinical aspects of cystic fibrosis in 35 patients. This paper was one of the earliest to recognize cystic fibrosis as a distinct clinical entity.

Dr. May is remembered as a very bright, outspoken and articulate person. He was a brilliant scientist and strove for the recognition of his Department. He was a scholar in the history of medicine and pediatrics. He was somewhat terse and quick thinking by nature and did not mince words; this personality trait led to some confrontations with persons in other Departments as well as within his own.

He is a member of the American Academy of Pediatrics, the Society for Pediatric Research and the American Pediatric Society. In 1950, he received the Mead-Johnson prize for his contributions on chronic nutritional disturbances in children. He served as editor of *Pediatrics* from 1954–1961.

PEDIATRIC FACULTY

During Dr. May's tenure as Department Head, several new faculty members were recruited. Dr. Robert Gauchat joined the Department as Chief Resident in 1952 after receiving an A.B. (1947) from Harvard College and his M.D. (1951) from Harvard Medical School. From 1951–52, he was a house officer at the University of Minnesota. From 1954–57, he was a Helen Hay Whitney Foundation Fellow in Pediatric Research. He joined the faculty at Iowa as Assistant Professor in 1955. His interests included cystic fibrosis and rheumatoid arthritis. He was keenly interested in the history of pediatrics and had an excellent library in the history of medicine. The collection of historic infant feeding devices he acquired is unique and extensive, and it now belongs to the American Academy of Pediatrics. It was on display at the University of Iowa Hospitals in 1985–1986. He was an excellent and demanding teacher and a superior clinician. He was to remain a member of the Department for the next 21 years, and was deeply involved in resident education.

Dr. Robert Jackson resigned from the Department in 1954 to become Chairman of the Department of Pediatrics at the University of Missouri, Columbia. He had been a popular professor in the College of Medicine, and many of the faculty had anticipated that he would be appointed to succeed Dr. Jeans as Head of the Department of Pediatrics. Relations between Dr. May and Dr. Jackson were strained during the two years that they served together in the Department before Dr. Jackson accepted the position at the University of Missouri. Coincident with the departure of Dr. Jackson in July 1954, Dr. Stearns left the Department of Pediatrics to join the faculty of the Department of Orthopedics. This left the management of the infant metabolic unit to Dr. May. Dr. Boyd resigned from the Department of Pediatrics effective July 1, 1952, when Dr. May arrived. An Assistant Professor, Dr. Roger Linke, also resigned from the Department at that time to pursue private practice in Minneapolis.

In July 1954 the pediatric faculty was reduced to three members: Dr. May, Dr. Floyd and Dr. MacQueen. However, during the summer and fall of that year Drs. Read, Fomon, Frazier, and Barnes joined the Department. Dr. Gauchat was chief resident in 1954–55 and joined the faculty as an Assistant Professor in 1955.

Dr. Samuel J. Fomon joined the faculty in 1954. He had received his B.A. from Harvard in 1945 and his M.D. from the University of Pennsylvania in 1947. He had interned at Queen's General Hospital 1947–48 and completed his residency in pediatrics at Children's Hospital of Philadelphia 1948–50. He did post-doctoral training in renal physiology at Cincinnati Cildren's Hospital Research Foundation from 1950–52. He was recruited by Dr. May to teach in the area of fluid and electrolyte balance and to set up a clinical research activity concerning patients with renal disease. However, soon after he arrived at Iowa and had established a laboratory to support the clinical research, Dr. May requested that he assume responsibility for the metabolic unit. Dr. Howard Meredith of the Iowa Child Welfare Research Station served as a tutor in anthropometry to Dr. Fomon and Dr. Fomon's research assistant, Mr. Ronald R. Rogers.

The metabolic unit at the time had a census of nine infants and a nursing staff consisting of Mrs. Thomas, five other nurses, and a nurse's aide. Drs. May and Fomon and Mrs. Thomas undertook a series of studies aimed at determining the requirement of infants for protein; and in 1958 Dr. May, partially on the basis of these studies, received the Borden Award of the American Academy of Pediatrics. Dr. Fomon continues his research of nutrition of infants and children today and is widely recognized as a leader in this field.

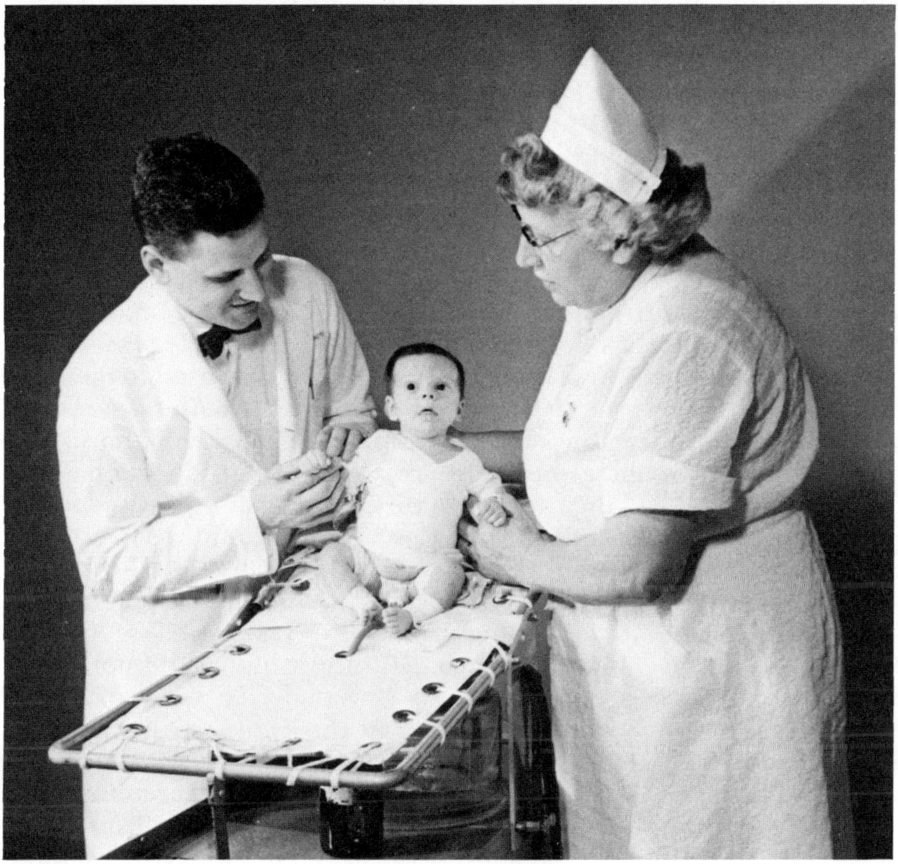

Samuel Fomon and Lora Thomas shown with a male infant on a metabolic bed.

During the chairmanship of Dr. May, Drs. Henry G. Cramblett, George M. Owen, and George T. Bryan were house officers. Dr. Cramblett subsequently joined the faculty of the University of Iowa and was the first virologist in Pediatrics, using tissue culture techniques. He later moved to Bowman Gray College of Medicine and then to the Ohio State University, where he served for some years in the Department of Microbiology and as Dean of the College of Medicine. Dr. Bryan received postdoctoral training in endocrinology under the supervision of Dr. Read and then joined the faculty of the University of Texas, Galveston, where he progressed to Professor of Pediatrics and then to Dean of the College of Medicine. Dr. Owen spent two years in postdoctoral training at the National Institutes of Health, then returned for a fellowship with Dr. Fomon and subsequently joined the faculty of the College of Medicine. He and Dr. Fomon worked together in renal studies, metabolic studies, and studies of growth and body composition.

Dr. Charles Read also joined the faculty in 1954. He received his M.D. from McGill University, Montreal, in 1943 and interned at the Royal Victoria Hospital, Montreal. From 1943–46, he served in the Royal Canadian Navy and from 1946–47 was a pediatric resident at Children's Memorial Hospital in Montreal. He was a pediatric fellow at Children's Memorial Hospital in Montreal from 1947–1949. He completed a fellowship in pediatric endocrinology from 1947–51 at Children's Memorial Hospital and Massachusetts General Hospital in Boston, where he was a Commonwealth Fellow. He was on the faculty of the University of Manitoba from 1951–54 before coming to Iowa. His early research included developing the first immunoassay, which was used to measure human growth hormone (1958). He pioneered in treating thyrotoxic children and adolescents with radioiodine. His instructional program for children with diabetes mellitus has served a vital educational role for these children and their families. He is a member of the Endocrine Society, the Society for Pediatric Research, the Midwest Pediatric Society, and the American Diabetes Society and organized the Iowa Affiliate of the American Diabetes Society, serving as president.

Dr. Robert Frazier joined the faculty in 1954. He received his B.S. and M.D. from the University of Chicago. His internship was completed at Yale University School of Medicine 1947–48 under Dr. Grover Powers. He was assistant resident in Pediatrics at the University of Colorado 1950–52 under Dr. Lubchenco. Before coming to Iowa, he was Instructor in Pediatrics at the University of Colorado. His research interests included cystic fibrosis and methods of its diagnosis. After leaving the Department in 1958, he became deeply involved in the activities of the American Academy of Pediatrics and served as its Executive Director from 1976–80.

Other faculty members joining the Department during Dr. May's tenure include Dr. George Barnes, who came in 1954. He was a spectacular teacher of pediatrics and was sought after as a pediatrician for the children of house staff and faculty members. He later left the Department to devote himself to radiology full time. Dr. Robert Kugel joined the Department in 1956 and helped organize the Child Development Program. Vinton Rowley, Ph.D., joined the Pediatric faculty in Child Psychology in 1957.

PHYSICAL PLANT

Dr. May wisely believed that the Department of Pediatrics could not expand or become a modern department if it stayed in Children's Hospital, for it was too isolated from the mainstream of University Hospital medicine. He devoted much effort toward moving the Department into General Hospital and this task was completed in 1954 when Pediatrics moved to 1 West.(1) A new outpatient clinic building which contained a small auditorium was built; this building is now the Student Health area. Also in 1954, the Hospital School for Severely Handicapped Children was completed. The outpatient department moved to General Hospital in 1955. The Medical Research Center was completed in 1957 and the Infant Metabolic Unit moved from Children's Hospital to the third floor of the MRC.

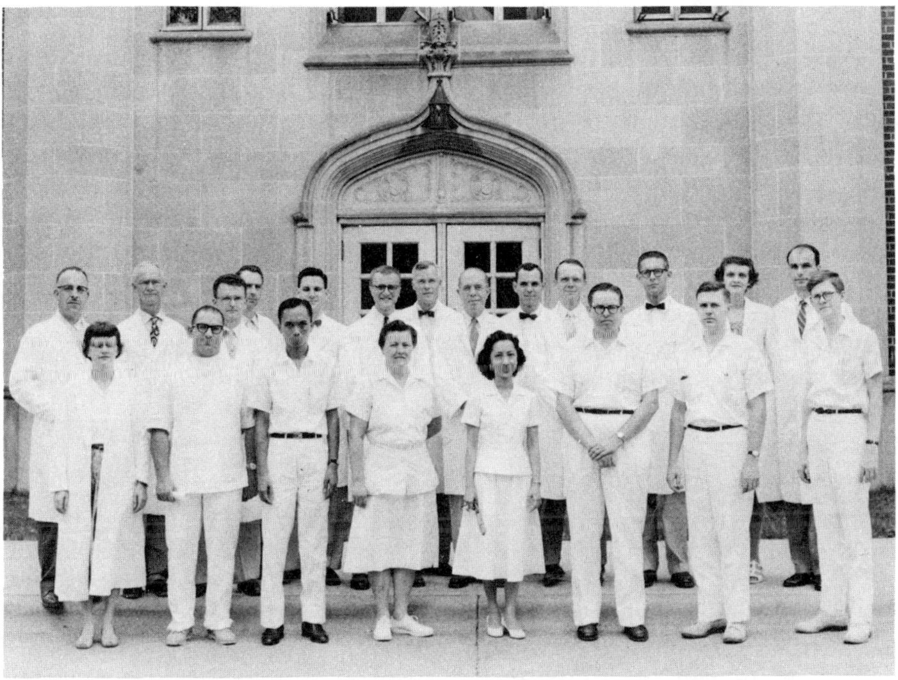

Pediatric faculty and staff, 1957–58. *Front row, left to right:* P. Cole, S. Nassif, R. de Guzman, D. Ehmke, L. Alejandrino, H. Cramblett, G. Owen, G. Bryan. *Second row, left to right:* R. Remboldt, M. Floyd, J. MacQueen, B. Goerlich, S. Fomon, W. Anderson, C. Read, C. May, G. Barnes, R. Kugel, R. Gauchat, P. Stivrins, R. Frazier.

RESIDENCY PROGRAM

The residency training program continued much in the same fashion under Dr. May as it had in Dr. Jeans's time, with some modifications. Because of the busy clinical service that existed at this time, faculty members were on service at all times. Resident call quarters moved to quonset huts built on the west side of the General Hospital when the wards moved to General Hospital. During this time, Dr. May and Dr. William Bean of the Department of Internal Medicine held monthly combined Pediatric and Internal Medicine Grand Rounds to discuss patients of mutual interest to both Departments.(2) After the Department moved to the west wing of the General Hospital, pediatric cardiac clinics were conducted with the medical cardiologists, residents in pediatrics and the fellows and staff from thoracic and cardiovascular surgery.

DEPARTMENTAL RESEARCH

Dr. May's tenure was a time of transition for the Department of Pediatrics, and he helped strengthen the program in the scholarly sense, recruiting faculty with research interests. There was an increased emphasis on laboratory research. This post-World War II period was also a time of increased availability of government funds for research from the rapidly expanding National Institutes of Health. The work of Dr. Fomon and the Metabolic Unit included defining the amino acid requirements for infants and further elucidating the protein requirements for infants considering the biologic differences of cow's milk and human milk. The other research interests of the Department during this time have been outlined under the names of the various faculty members.

LATER ACCOMPLISHMENTS

Dr. May left Iowa in 1957 and served as Professor of Pediatrics at New York University from 1957 to 1970. He became Executive Director of the Physicians Council for Information on Child Health in 1957. In 1970, he became a Professor of Pediatrics at the University of Colorado and he has maintained a subspecialty interest in pediatric allergy, especially food allergy. He is currently retired and living in Vermont. After Dr. May left, Dr. MacQueen served as acting chairman until Dr. Wallace McCrory came as Department Head in 1958.

References

1 Personal communication: Dr. John MacQueen.

2 Personal communication: Dr. William Bean.

WALLACE W. McCRORY
1958–1961

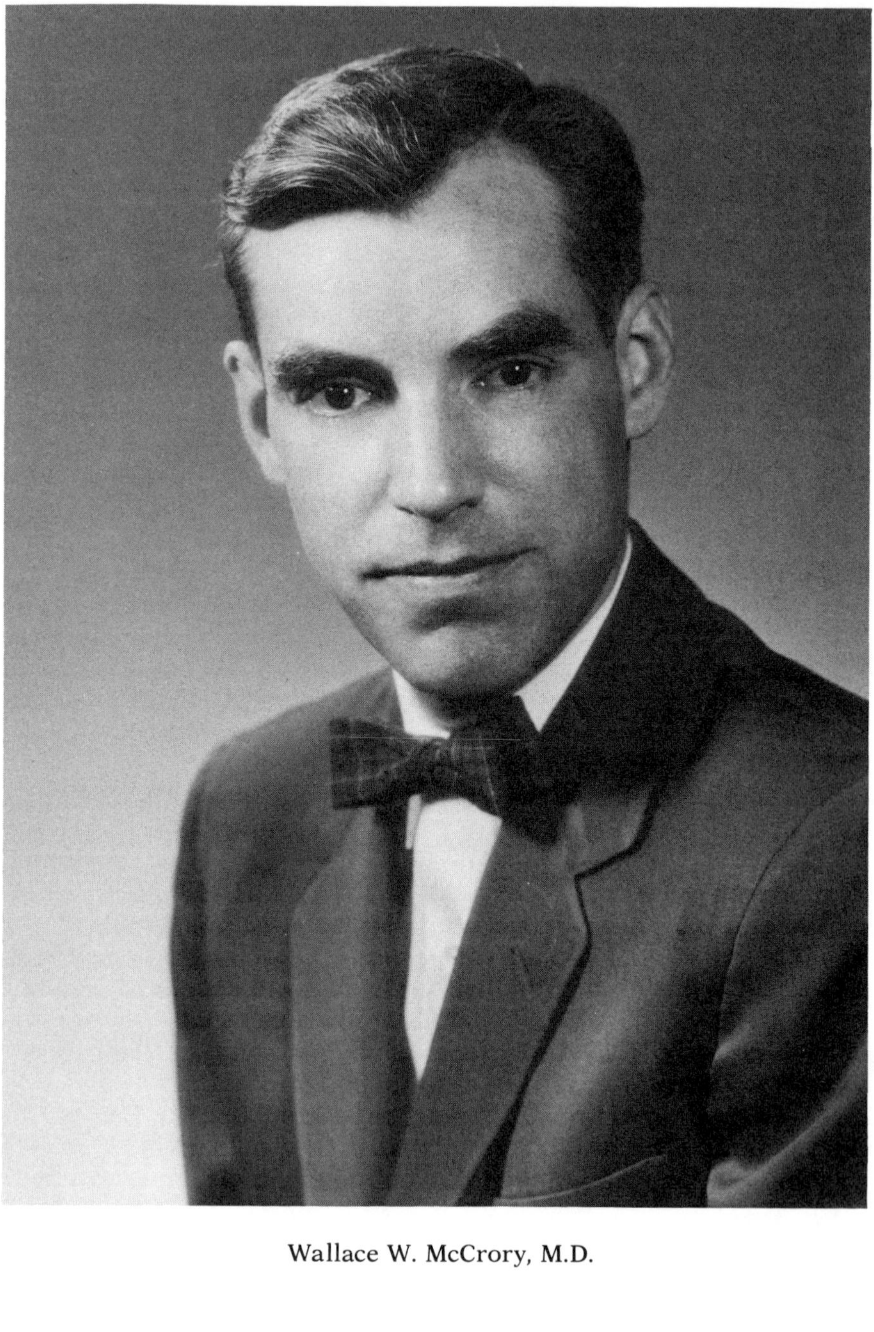

Wallace W. McCrory, M.D.

WALLACE W. McCRORY

Dr. McCrory was born in 1920. He studied at the University of Wisconsin earning a B.S. in 1941 and an M.D. in 1944. He was a rotating intern at Philadelphia General Hospital (1944–45) and was then a Pediatric Resident (1945–46) and Chief Resident (1948–49) at Children's Hospital of Philadelphia. He was a Lewis Cass Ledyard Jr. Research Fellow in Pediatrics at Cornell, N.Y. Hospital 1949–50. From 1950 to 1958, he successively served as Assistant Professor and Associate Professor of Pediatrics at the University of Pennsylvania School of Medicine. His area of special interest was pediatric nephrology. His professional affiliations include the American Academy of Pediatrics, the Society for Pediatric Research, Alpha Omega Alpha, and the American Pediatric Society. On coming to Iowa, he sought to develop further pediatric subspecialties and stronger fellowship training programs and to increase both clinical and laboratory research.

PEDIATRIC FACULTY

At the time of Dr. McCrory's arrival, the core faculty was composed of Drs. MacQueen, Rembolt, Floyd, Fomon, Read, Cramblett, Gauchat, Barnes and Kugel. Three faculty members of note joined the Department during his chairmanship.

Dr. Robert Carter joined the faculty in 1959 and was the first pediatric hematologist/oncologist at Iowa. He became Assistant Dean of the College of Medicine in 1962.

Dr. Johannes (Hans) Zellweger was recruited to join the faculty by Dean Nelson of the College of Medicine at the time Dr. May was leaving, and arrived during Dr. McCrory's tenure. His career before coming to Iowa was noteworthy. He graduated from Zurich Medical School in 1934 and completed a pediatric residency at Kantonspital, Lucern, Switzerland, 1934–37. From 1937 to 1939, he worked in the Hospital of Dr. Albert Schweitzer. He had further pediatric training at Children's Hospital, Zurich, Switzerland, from 1940 to 1951 where he worked with Dr. Guido Fanconi. From 1951 to 1959, he was Head of the Pediatric Department at the American University of Beirut before coming the Iowa in 1959. He is a superb clinician, a true gentleman, and a renowned dysmorphologist. His research interests are many, including neuromuscular diseases, human genetics and cytogentics and he is the author of numerous publications.

Dr. Jacqueline Noonan became the first trained pediatric cardiologist at Iowa when she joined the Department in 1959, coming from Boston. Her subspecialty training and diagnostic expertise permitted patients who had previously been followed by Internal Medicine to receive general pediatric and subspecialty care in the Pediatric Department. During her tenure at Iowa from 1958 to 1961, she also trained the first fellow in pediatric cardiology at Iowa, Dr. Dorothy Ehmke. Dr. Noonan helped organize the field clinics in cardiology and the cardiology clinics at University Hospital.

Dr. McCrory, whose area of interest was renal disease, established the Pediatric Nephrology Division at Iowa.

PHYSICAL PLANT

There were no major changes in the physical plant during Dr. McCrory's tenure. The Child Development Clinic opened in 1958 to serve as a diagnostic clinic for developmental, learning and behavior problems in children. In 1960, the chromosome lab was opened by Dr. Zellweger, assisted by Dr. John Opitz, who was then a resident in the Department. During Dr. McCrory's tenure, the Department of Pediatrics assumed professional responsibility for the management of the Newborn Nursery. This had previously been the responsibility of the Department of Obstetrics.

RESIDENCY PROGRAM

The residency training program had an international flavor during Dr. McCrory's chairmanship, since many of the residents were from countries such as Argentina, Columbia, Iran, Lebanon, Phillipines, Germany, Iceland, Belgium, Turkey, and Bolivia. Dr. Ehmke completed her pediatric residency and began her pediatric cardiology fellowship during this period. Dr. John Opitz was also a resident in pediatrics during Dr. McCrory's chairmanship. Dr. Hugh Moffet, now at the University of Wisconsin, was also a resident at this time. Residents were on call every other night and call quarters remained in the quonset huts on the west side of the General Hospital. These communal quarters were flimsily constructed and were shared with ants and rodents.(1) Dr. Gauchat was always involved in resident and student education.

DEPARTMENTAL RESEARCH

Drs. Read, Fomon, Cramblett and Gauchat continued the research they were involved in during Dr. May's chairmanship. Dr. Noonan and Dr. Ehmke published an article describing the children with characteristic dysmorphic features and cardiac findings of what is now known as the

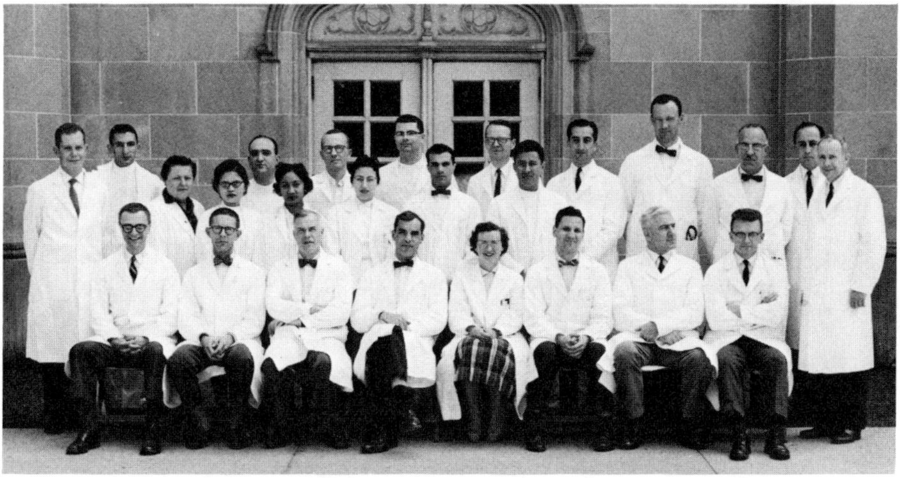

Pediatric faculty and house staff, 1959–60. *First row, left to right:* Drs. W. B. Anderson, R. D. Gauchat, C. H. Read, W. W. McCrory, J. A. Noonan, S. J. Fomon, H. Zellweger, J. C. MacQueen. *Second row:* Drs. D. A. Ehmke, M. Grino, M. Pine, N. Haddad, H. Naficy, J. Merida. *Third row:* Drs. G. H. Fleischaker, K. Naficy, M. Cusminsky, G. Porter, H. Moffet, R. B. Kugel, S. Najjar, R. E. Carter, R. R. Remboldt, M. Bingol, T. Alexander.

Noonan-Ehmke Syndrome. Dr. Zellweger published several articles related to clinical genetics research.

LATER ACCOMPLISHMENTS

Dr. McCrory left the University of Iowa in 1961 to become Chairman of the Department of Pediatrics at Cornell University in New York, a position he held until 1980. He is currently Pediatrician-in-Chief and Director of Nephrology at Cornell and is a member of the American Society of Nephrology and the American Society of Pediatric Nephrology. In addition, he has served on the editorial board of the Pediatrics Review and Education Program.

Reference

1 Personal communication: Dr. John Opitz.

DONAL DUNPHY
1961–1973

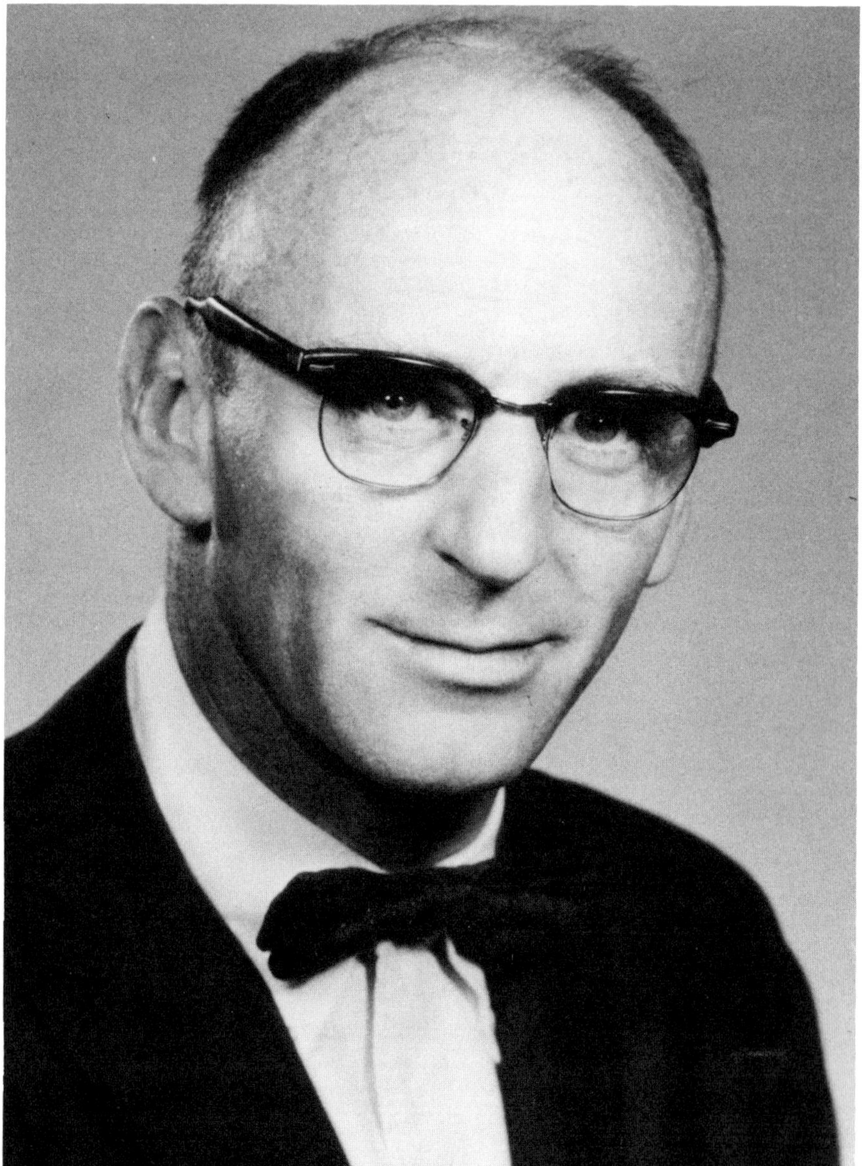

Donal Dunphy, M.D.

DONAL DUNPHY

Dr. Donal Dunphy was born in 1917 in Northhampton, Massachusetts. He received his B.A. in 1939 from Holy Cross College and his M.D. in 1944 from Yale University. He completed his internship and residency from 1943–1946 at New Haven General Hospital. During his residency he and another house officer, Dr. Robert Cook, were the first to use streptomycin in the treatment of a human. An infant with tuberculous meningitis was treated with streptomycin and was the first reported recovery from what was then a uniformly fatal disease. Dr. Dunphy's early work was in infectious disease, including the development of simple media for culture of the tubercle bacillus.

From 1947 to 1950, he was an Instructor in Pediatrics at Yale University School of Medicine and he then completed a parttime fellowship in Pediatric Cardiology from 1950 to 1953, again at Yale. He then was in private pediatric practice for three years in Stratford, Connecticut and worked with Dr. Richard Olmsted who was later Head of Pediatrics at the University of Oregon. From 1953 to 1955, Dr. Dunphy served in the Army. From 1955 to 1961, he successively served as Associate, Assistant Professor and Associate Professor in Pediatrics at Buffalo Children's Hospital, Buffalo, N.Y. He then came to Iowa, in 1961, as Professor and Head of the Department of Pediatrics.

Those who worked with Dr. Dunphy remember him as a very intelligent and dedicated teacher. He was a kind and gentle physician who was loved by his patients and was an excellent clinician and speaker. He loved teaching and devoted tremendous effort to resident education. As a consequence, he actively recruited several new clinical faculty members and strove to improve resident recruiting. Also, he had a delightful sense of humor and was often called "the last of the practical jokers."

He is a member of several societies including the American Academy of Pediatrics, New York Academy of Science, American Pediatric Society and the American Medical Association. He served as the Director of the Child Development Study at Buffalo Children's Hospital from 1955–1959 and was Director of an National Institutes of Health Collaborative project there from 1958–1961. He served as pediatric consultant to the National Institute of Neurologic Disease and Blindness from 1960–1961.

PEDIATRIC FACULTY

Donal Dunphy made several lasting contributions to the Department of Pediatrics at Iowa. He sought to improve pediatric teaching and clinical services and also to improve the resident education program. As he worked towards these goals he recruited several excellent new faculty members. When Dr. Dunphy arrived in 1961, the core pediatric faculty consisted of Drs. Floyd, Fomon, Gauchat, Kugel, MacQueen, Noonan, Read, Remboldt and Zellweger. All told, there were 13 senior staff members in Pediatrics in 1961.

Dr. James Taylor joined the faculty in 1961. He was very active in clinical practice and resident teaching during his time at Iowa. He was in charge of the Pediatric Hematology/Oncology Service along with Dr. Andre Lascari, who joined the Department in 1966. Together they supervised the treatment of childhood cancer in the Department. Dr. Taylor's tragic death in 1976 was felt by all members of the Pediatric Department. His teaching skill is remembered each year with the James Taylor Teacher of the Year Award.

Dr. Gerald Solomons came in 1962 to head the Child Development Clinic (CDC), after leaving an appointment in the Institute of Health Sciences at Brown University, Providence, Rhode Island. He advanced to Professor of Pediatrics in 1969 and was director of the CDC until his

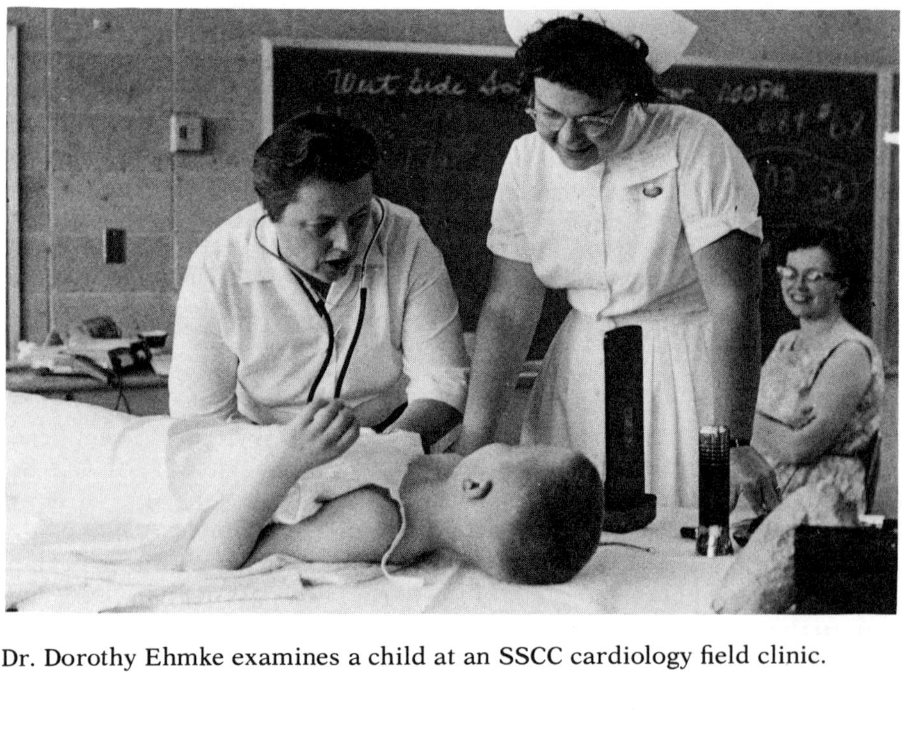

Dr. Dorothy Ehmke examines a child at an SSCC cardiology field clinic.

retirement in 1985. In addition, he was active in research and teaching related to child abuse.

Dr. Dorothy Ehmke, Ph.D., M.D., completed her cardiology fellowship in 1962 and joined the faculty as an Associate. Jacqueline Noonan left in 1962 to become Director of the Pediatric Cardiology Section of the University of Kentucky at Lexington. In her absence, Drs. Ehmke and Dunphy remained as pediatric cardiologists until Dr. Peter Vlad came in 1963. Dr. Ehmke assumed the role of supervisor of the SSCC Cardiology Field Clinics and played an active role in medical student, resident, and fellow education in cardiology.

Dr. Peter Vlad joined the Department in 1963 to head the Division of Pediatric Cardiology. His circuitous route in coming to Iowa City was an interesting one. He was Rumanian, and in that country his family name is associated with Count Vlad, better known as "Count Dracula." Dr. Vlad fled the country on foot at the end of World War II and went to Paris. There he worked with Dr. Soulie, an eminent French cardiologist who did much to describe the pathology of congenital heart disease. From Paris, he went to Toronto, Canada, and worked with Dr. Keith Rowe. Together they wrote one of the first textbooks on pediatric cardiology. From Toronto, he went to Buffalo Children's Hospital to work in pediatric cardiology before coming to Iowa. While in Toronto he was both a medical student and a member of the teaching faculty because of licensing requirements. His arrival in Iowa brought major developments in cardiology to Pediatrics and Internal Medicine. He brought great expertise in cardiac catheterization and reorganized the cath labs for Pediatrics and Internal Medicine. At this time, both labs were located on the third floor of General Hospital. He was the first person at Iowa and one of the first in the world to perform left heart catheterization. This revolutionized the study of left heart disease. As a physician, he was an outspoken and notable figure. He smoked cigars while making ward rounds and his somewhat argumentative nature brought him into conflict with the Chief of Thoracic and Cardiovascular Surgery more than once. Dr. Vlad remained on the faculty until his resignation in 1968.(1)

Dr. William E. Bell joined the Pediatric faculty in 1963. He received his M.D. from the Medical College of Virginia in 1955. He completed his residency in neurology at the University of Iowa from 1955 to 1959, followed by a fellowship in pediatric neurology at Iowa from 1962–63. He is board-certified in neurology and pediatrics, and holds a special certificate in child neurology. His areas of clinical research include increased intracranial pressure, CNS infections, perinatal and neonatal hypoxic and ischemic brain lesions and intracranial neoplasms in childhood. He is widely admired as a general pediatrician and pediatric neurologist, and plays an active role in medical student and resident teaching. He is the author of numerous publications, textbook chapters, and is co-author of the texts *Increased Intracranial Pressure in Children* and *Neurologic Infections in Childhood.*

Dr. Lloyd J. Filer, Jr., received a Ph.D. degree in biochemistry at the University of Pittsburgh in 1944, an M.D. degree at the University of Rochester in 1952 and soon thereafter became Medical Director of Ross Laboratories, where, among his many other activites, he carried out a nutrition research program with piglets. In 1965, when Ross Laboratories became a subsidiary of Abbott Laboratories, Dr. Filer's research opportunities were greatly diminished and he resigned from his position to join the faculty of the University of Iowa, where he and Dr. Fomon worked collaboratively with both human infants and miniature pigs. In addition to his involvement in resident education, his research interests are many and include metabolic studies in infants, placental transfer of nutrients, food additives, and total parental nutrition. He became Professor Emeritus in Pediatrics in 1986.

Dr. Thomas A. Anderson received a Ph.D. degree in nutritional biochemistry at the University of Arizona, served on the faculty of the University of South Dakota and then served as Director of Nutritional Research at the H. J. Heinz Company, before joining the faculty of the University of Iowa in 1970. He collaborated with Drs. Fomon and Filer in a number of studies of human infants and piglets and later carried out nutritional studies of newborn rat pups. He retired in 1984.

In 1961, Dr. Fomon received a Career Development Award from the National Institutes of Health. By that time he had become so engrossed in his work in nutrition, growth and body composition that he turned over the renal service to Dr. Owen and a postdoctoral trainee, Dr. Carl E. Nelsen, who subsequently joined the faculty. In 1965, Dr. Owen accepted a position as Medical Director of Bristol-Myers International.

Also in 1965, Lewis D. Stegink, Ph.D., became a faculty member. His area of expertise is biochemistry and in addition to overseeing the operation of the amino acid laboratory, he has several areas of research, including the biochemical changes occuring during abnormal and normal development of the infant, amino acid toxicity, placental transfer of amino acids, and infant and post-surgical nutrition.

Dr. Sidney Kripke joined the Department in 1966 and was involved in the development of the ambulatory pediatric program. In addition, he helped start the pediatric nurse practitioner program at Iowa. He was extensively involved in resident and medical teaching. Dr. Dave Silber was also active in the Ambulatory Division.

George Baker, M.D., became a member of the Pediatric faculty as an Instructor in 1964. He was the first neonatologist in the Department and in 1968, organized the neonatal transport van service to facilitate transfer of sick neonates to the University Hospital. He has always been dedicated to medical education and in 1970 became an Assistant Dean in the College of Medicine.

James Hardy, Ph.D., joined the faculty in 1966 as Associate Professor of Speech Pathology and was also the Director of the Speech and Hearing Clinic in the Department of Speech Pathology and Audiology. He has been active in the clinical aspects of his field at Hospital School and has been involved in research involving normal speech breathing physiology and its aberrations in many neuromuscular disorders. He later became Director of Professional Services for the Division of Developmental Disabilities.

Dr. Robert Durnin served on the faculty in the Division of Pediatric Cardiology from 1967–1971. Another faculty member in Cardiology during this time was Dr. Chandramouli, who completed his Fellowship in Pediatric Cardiology here from 1966–1968. He became an Associate in Pediatric Cardiology in 1972 and currently practices in Des Moines, Iowa.

Dr. Alfred Healy joined the Pediatric faculty in 1967 and became Associate Medical Director of the University Hospital School. In addition to his responsibilities at Hospital School, he has been active in resident teaching and recruitment. He became Medical Director of Hospital School in 1977.

Charles F. Johnson, M.D., joined the Department in 1968. He was involved in the operation of the Child Development Clinic and medical student and resident teaching. He left the Department in 1977.

James Stehbens, Ph.D., joined the faculty in 1967 in Pediatric Psychology and has been interested in the psychological consequences of premature and other high risk pregnancies. He has also been actively involved in research involving the oncology patients and their families.

Ronald Lauer, M.D., came to Iowa in 1968 to head the Division of Pediatric Cardiology when Dr. Vlad left. He received his M.D. from the University of Manitoba in 1953 and interned at Winnipeg General Hospital, 1953–1954. He then did residency training in pediatrics in Canada, England and the United States before beginning his fellowship in pediatric cardiology. He studied pediatric cardiology successively at Buffalo Children's Hospital, the Mayo Clinic and the Hospital for Sick Children in Toronto. He held faculty appointments at the University of Kansas before coming to Iowa. Under his direction, the Division of Pediatric Cardiology has been active in research, teaching and patient care, achieving national prominence.

Victor Ionasescu, M.D., joined the faculty in 1968. A native of Rumania, he received his M.D. and did his residency in Bucharest. He later studied neurology and genetics in Rumania, Italy and Switzerland before coming to Iowa. His areas of interest include clinical genetics and the biochemistry of neuromuscular disorders.

Dr. Ekhard E. Ziegler was born in Austria, received his M.D. degree from the University of Innsbruck, and carried out some research there before arriving at the University of Iowa for postdoctoral training in nutrition. Upon completion of his training in 1970, he returned to Austria; but in 1973 he was appointed to the faculty of the University of Iowa. He joined Dr. Fomon in nutritonal studies of term infants, but also obtained training in neonatology and has subsequently pursued nutritional questions both of term and preterm infants.

Carl Betts, Ph.D., has been actively involved in the speech and hearing problems of children since he received his M.A. in 1955. He earned his Ph.D. in 1963 and has been involved with the Child Development Clinic, Hospital School, and the SSCC Clinics for which he has been Director of Speech and Hearing Services.

Linda Rames, M.D., served on the faculty of Pediatrics from 1970 to 1977. Her subspecialty interest was nephrology, and she was involved in the clinical nephrology service and resident and medical student teaching.

M. Kabir Younoszai, M.D., became a faculty member in Pediatrics in 1970 after completing his fellowship in gastroenterology at Iowa. His M.D. and internship were completed at the American University of Beirut. He has headed the Division of Gastroenterology since its start in 1970.

Dr. Brenda Cruikshank joined the faculty of Pediatrics in 1970 and has been active in Ambulatory Pediatrics and the Pediatric Nurse Practitioner Program. Dr. Mary Waziri also became a faculty member in 1970, and has been working in the Division of Medical Genetics.

Lee Forrest Hill, M.D., former Chief of Pediatrics and Director of Pediatric Education at Raymond Blank Memorial Hospital for Children in Des Moines, formed a long and productive relationship with the University of Iowa during Dr. Dunphy's tenure. From 1961 to 1971 he was a Clinical Professor of Pediatrics at the University. He commuted to Iowa City once weekly to attend the child health and ambulatory pediatrics clinics. In the 1960s he was instrumental in developing an off-campus clinical clerkship in pediatrics for University of Iowa students in Des Moines. He was an extremely bright and caring practitioner and teacher of pediatrics who had a rare ability to combine successfully a place in both academia and private practice. He served as American Academy of Pediatrics District Chairman 1941–1945 and as AAP President 1946–1947. He was awarded the Academy's Grulee Medal for Service to Pediatrics in 1952. In addition, he served as president of the American Board of Pediatrics longer than any other and served on the editorial board of the *Journal of Pediatrics* for more than 25 years. In recognition of his many contributions to pediatric education, he was elected to membership in the American Pediatric Society. He died in 1980.(2)

Jack Spevak, M.D., a general pediatrician and pediatric hematologist/oncologist from Des Moines was a member of the clinical teaching faculty from 1963 to 1967. In addition, he taught at Raymond Blank

Memorial Hospital, where he was in charge of pediatric education and was Professor and Chairman of Pediatrics at the College of Osteopathic Medicine in Des Moines from 1972 to 1975.

PHYSICAL PLANT

During Dr. Donal Dunphy's tenure as Department Head the pediatric wards initially occupied the 1 West area of General Hospital. The adolescent ward was opened on 5 South in 1967 and was moved to 2 West in 1970. The first infant intensive care unit with cardiorespiratory monitors and ventilators at Iowa opened in 1W 104 in 1968 with four beds and was later expanded to six beds. An intensive care lab was built nearby to provide around the clock microchemistry laboratory service. The Pediatric Outpatient area was expanded and remodeled in 1972. In 1974, a new Pediatric Cardiology area was built and housed the new cardiac cath lab. This was built with the money from the Hill-Burton Foundation. An addition was made to the Hospital School with federal funds. This unit was designed to provide physical space for the cytogenetics laboratory, neuropathology research and a biochemical laboratory to support these programs in Nutrition. It also housed the Child Development facilities.

RESIDENCY PROGRAM

Dr. Dunphy devoted much thought and effort to the improvement of the residency program. When he came in 1961, the housestaff consisted of nine residents. He was actively involved in resident teaching and sought faculty members who also would be. During his tenure, the clinical services in Pediatrics were improved and the residency program grew to be a respected one. When he stepped down as Chairman in 1972, there were twenty-one residents.

DEPARTMENTAL GROWTH AND RESEARCH

When Dr. Dunphy came on staff in 1961, there were 13 senior staff on the Pediatric faculty; and in 1972, there were 35. The growth of the Department during this time was especially strong in the areas of clinical services and he divided the Department into various divisions for administrative purposes. The SSCC Field Clinics were increased in number and scope during this time under the leadership of Dr. John MacQueen working in collaboration with the Department and Dr. Dunphy. The research activities of the Department were mainly in the field of nutrition as well as clinical and psychologically oriented studies.

Dr. Dunphy decided to resign as Department Head in 1971, but served until replaced by Dr. Fred G. Smith in 1973. He left Iowa City in 1973

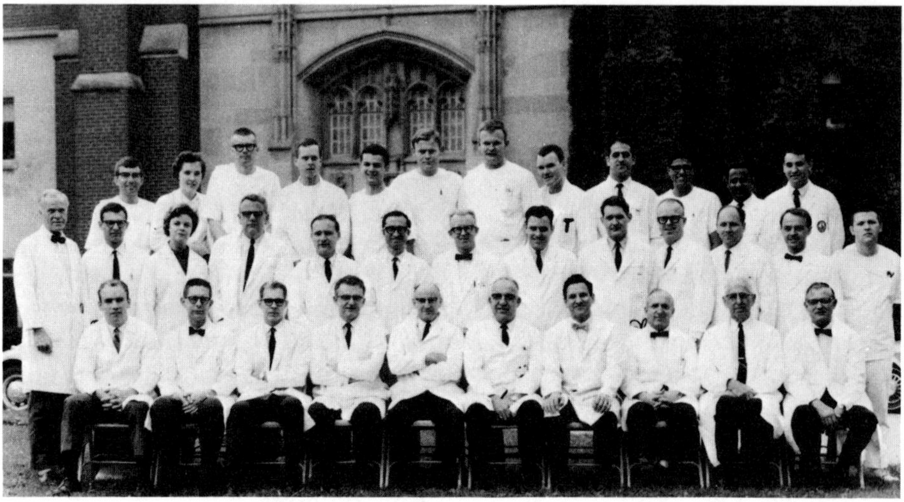

Pediatric house staff and faculty, 1967–68. *First row* (*seated*): J. Stehbens, R. Gauchat, W. Bell, J. MacQueen, D. Dunphy, R. Remboldt, S. Fomon, G. Solomons, L. F. Hill, L. J. Filer. *Second row:* C. Read, S. Kripke, J. Anderson, V. Rowley, A. Healey, C. Johnson, G. Normanly, G. Alley, R. Durnin, L. Stegink, A. Lascari, G. Baker, C. Putman. *Third row:* H. Schneider, E. Riegle, J. Ziska, P. Roseboom, A. Balanoff, C. Smith, D. Tweito, W. McAveney, R. Hawit, Z. Lababidi, B. Chandramouli, J. Scheinman.

and moved to the University of North Carolina to head the pediatric section of the Area Health Education Center program. This is a program designed to involve all of the schools in the Health Science Campus in statewide education programs, including the development of 300 new primary care resident positions in nine different centers. He is a member of the American Board of Pediatrics and served as Vice President. He is a member of the American Board of Family Medicine, the Residency Review Committee for Pediatrics and its current Chairperson.

References

1 Personal communication: Dr. Ronald Lauer.

2 Nelson WE. And the walls come tumbling down: A tribute to Lee Forrest Hill. J Ped 1976; 89:1–2.

FRED G. SMITH, JR.
1973–1986

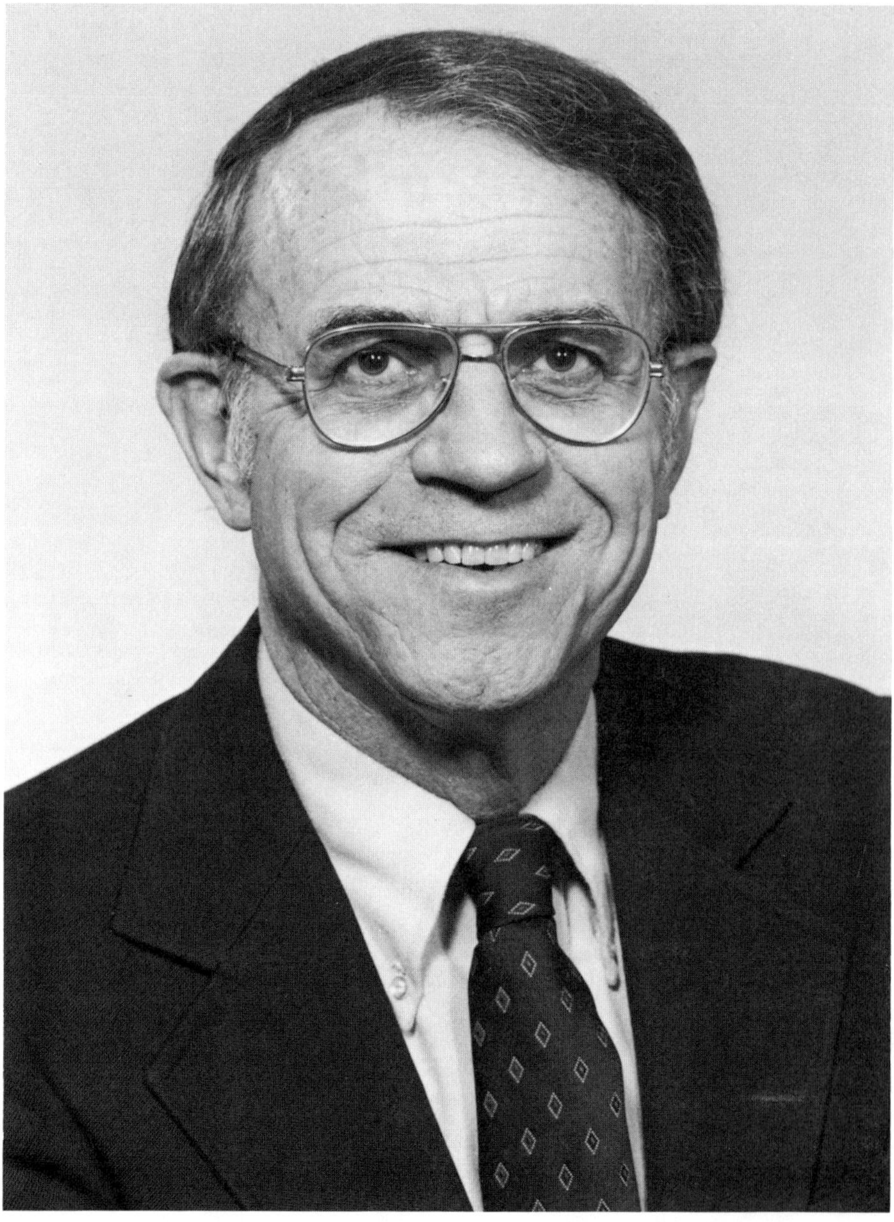

Fred G. Smith, Jr., M.D.

FRED G. SMITH, JR.

Fred G. Smith, Jr. was born in 1928. He received his B.S. from UCLA in 1951 and his M.D. from UCLA in 1955. He completed his internship at UCLA in 1955–1956. Following this he continued his pediatric residency and also completed a pediatric nephrology fellowship at the University of Minnesota Hospital from 1956–1957. He returned to UCLA from 1957–1958 where he was resident and chief resident in pediatrics. His academic appointments began with his assignment to the 1604th U.S.A.F. Hospital as Chief of Pediatrics and outpatient clinics from 1958–1960. From 1960 to 1973 he advanced from Assistant Professor to Professor of Pediatrics at UCLA. In addition, he was director of the residency training program at UCLA from 1964 to 1966 and Chief of the Division of Pediatric Nephrology from 1966 to 1971. In 1968–1969 he was a U.S.P.H.S. special research fellow at St. Mary's Hospital in London, England. He was appointed Professor and Head of Pediatrics at the University of Iowa in 1973.

Dr. Smith is an exceptionally dedicated pediatric educator and practitioner. He is respected as a nephrologist as well as a general pediatrician. His warm and caring attitude towards patients and their families is readily evident. He has repeatedly shown his commitment to resident education and Departmental development in areas of clinical services, teaching and research.

The professional affiliations of Dr. Smith are many and include the American Board of Pediatrics, the American Academy of Pediatrics, the Society for Pediatric Research, the American Pediatric Society, and the American Society of Pediatric Nephrology. His research interests have been primarily in fetal physiology and developmental nephrology.

PEDIATRIC FACULTY AND RESEARCH

Since the time of Dr. Smith's arrival in 1973, the Department has witnessed a remarkable period of growth and development paralleling that of the field of pediatrics itself. The advances in the Department have included faculty recruitment, teaching, clinical services, research, resident education, and growth of the physical plant.

When Dr. Smith became Department Head there were 39 senior staff members in Pediatrics. There has subsequently been tremendous growth in the size and depth of the faculty with enlargement of the divisions created by Dr. Dunphy and the addition of several new divisions.

Since his arrival, he has sought to establish and maintain a core of faculty who would in turn aid in the recruitment of new faculty and in the perpetuation of Departmental research. Early additions to the faculty included Dr. C. Thomas Kisker (Hematology/ Oncology), Dr. Robert J. Roberts (Pharmacology, Neonatology), Dr. Richard Schieken (Cardiology), and Dr. Herman Hein (Neonatology), all in 1973. The following year further additions included Dr. Allen Erenberg (Neonatology), Dr. Robert G. Thompson (Endocrinology), Dr. Martin Meyers (Infectious Disease), and Dr. Jean Robillard (Nephrology).

The growth of the various Departmental divisions and the development of new divisions has been substantial. Currently there are 18 divisions in Pediatrics including: Allergy/Pulmonary, Ambulatory, Biochemistry, Cardiology, Developmental Disabilities, Endocrinology, Gastroenterology, Genetics, Hematology/Oncology, Infectious Disease, Neonatology, Nephrology, Neurology, Nutrition, Clinical Pharmacology and Toxicology, Psychology, Speech and Hearing, and Child Health Specialty Clinics.

The Division of Pediatric Infectious Diseases was organized in 1974 when Dr. Martin Meyers joined the faculty. He served as Division Head until he left in 1981 to join the faculty of Children's Hospital of Cincinnati. He was joined by Dr. Betty Edmond in 1980; and she served as acting Division Head until 1982, when she left to take a position at the Colorado Medical Center. Also, Dr. Donna Bosworth was a Division member from 1981–1982 and was very active in resident teaching. The current Division consists of Dr. Richard Andersen (1982), Dr. Stanley Perlman (1983) and Dr. Charles Grose (1984), Division Head. Their research interests involve the molecular biology of viruses, studying herpes simplex, varicella zoster and corona virus using molecular techniques.

The Division of Neonatology was formed in 1974 when Dr. Allen Erenberg became a faculty member. The growth of this Division has paralleled that of the specialty itself, which emerged only in the late 1960s. The first Neonatal ICU at Iowa opened in 1975 with 12 beds. Faculty in the Division include Dr. Herman Hein, Dr. Gail McGuinness (1977) and Dr. Edward Bell (1979). In addition, Dr. Robert Roberts of the Division of Pharmacology and Dr. Ekhard Ziegler of the Division of Nutrition are Division members. Dr. Kenneth Nakamura joined the Division in 1986, having completed a Fellowship in Neonatology and Pediatric residency at the University of Iowa. Research interests include perinatal health care delivery, neonatal pharmacology, developmental nephrology, oxygen toxicity, pulmonary injury in neonates, parenteral nutrition, thermoregulation, and pulmonary hypertension.

The Allergy and Pulmonary Division was created in 1975 with the addition of Dr. Miles Weinberger to the staff. Subsequently, Dr. Richard Ahrens and Dr. Jeffrey Wagener have joined the Division in 1980 and

1983, respectively. The Division's research has involved chiefly the pharmacotherapy of drugs used in the management of asthma. Studies have included theophylline pharmocotherapy, delivery and deposition of aerosolized drugs, and bronchial provocation examining the pharmacokinetics of inhaled bronchodilators. Dr. Wagener is studying lung growth and development using a fetal lamb model with altered pulmonary artery perfusion. The Cystic Fibrosis Center at The University of Iowa is directed by this Division. Dr. Wagener became medical director of the PICU in 1985 and also directs the operation of the Pediatric Pulmonary Function Laboratory.

The Division of Nephrology was formally organized by Dr. Smith. Dr. Robillard became Head of the Division of Nephrology in 1974 and is a recognized leader in fetal nephrology. Under his direction the Division has received national and international recognition for its research in developmental nephrology. Major contributions have been made to the understanding of renal development in the fetus and newborn, including the development of glomerular filtration; the role of hormonal control via aldosterone, vasopressin, and angiotension; and the development of sympathetic control of renal blood flow. Current members include Drs. Jean Robillard (1974), Doug Weismann (1977), and Jerold Woodhead (1979). Areas of research include a variety of studies in developmental nephrology and physiology, neonatal pharmacology, and chronic renal failure.

Dr. James Hanson, who joined the Department in 1976, currently heads the Division of Medical Genetics. He is joined by Drs. Hans Zellweger (1959), Victor Ionasescu (1968), Mary Waziri (1972), Shivanand Patil (1977), James Bartley (1979), William Rhead (1979), Jeffrey Murray (1984), and Wilma Krause (1985). The Division is involved in research including clinical genetics, teratology, organic acidemias, neuromuscular disease, cancer cytogenics, biochemical genetics, DNA sequencing, and genetic counseling. Dr. Patil supervises the operation of the cytogenetics laboratory. Dr. Krause directs the operation of the metabolic disease clinic. In addition to their work at the University Hospitals, they serve the state through the Regional Genetic Consultation Service.

The Division of Pediatric Endocrinology includes Drs. Charles Read (1954), Robert Thompson (1974), and Eva Tsalikian (1983). Dr. John Hayford was a member of the Department and this Division from 1977 until his untimely death in 1983; the John Hayford Pediatric Research Award for residents was created in his memory. Research interests of the Division include the treatment of thyrotoxicosis with radioiodine, dietary influence of lipid and carbohydrate homeostasis in the normal and diabetic child, and hormonal control of amino acid metabolism. Dr. Read retired in 1986, and Dr. Thompson resigned in August, 1986 to assume charge of growth hormone studies at Eli Lilly and Company.

The Pediatric Hematology and Oncology Division has grown substantially since Dr. Smith's arrival. Division members include Drs. C. Thomas Kisker (1974), Ronald Strauss (1976), Raymond Tannous (1977), Pedro deAlarcon (1983), Roger Giller (1983), and Michael Trigg (1986). Jack Spevak, M.D., was a Division member from 1977 to 1981 and was widely admired as a teacher, advisor, and clinician. The Division is a member of the Children's Cancer Study Group and directs a center for treatment of hemophilia. In addition to its activities within Pediatrics, the Division holds conferences with the Departments of Pathology and Internal Medicine. Research interests are many and include evaluating systems of health care delivery to children with hematologic and oncologic diseases in their local communities. Additional areas of research include leukocyte physiology and function, bone marrow transplantation, leukophoresis and granulocyte transfusions, blood coagulation in the fetus, and platelet recovery following bone marrow transplantation. Dr. Strauss became medical director of the Elmer DeGowin Blood Center in 1983. Dr. Trigg directs the five-bed Pediatric Bone Marrow Transplantation Unit on 7 Carver East.

The Division of Pediatric Cardiology maintains an extremely busy inpatient and outpatient service and has grown substantially since 1973. Dr. Ronald Lauer heads the Division. Other faculty members include Drs. William Marvin (1979), Edward Clark (1980), Julia Lee (1980), Larry Mahoney (1982), Diane Atkins (1984), Ming Young (1985), and Michael Florentine (1985). Dr. Richard Schieken was a Division member from 1973 to 1981. Dr. Dorothy Ehmke retired in 1983 after more than twenty years of service. The Division directs the cardiac catheterization and electrophysiology laboratory. Research interests of the Division include the epidemiology of hypertension and arteriosclerosis in childhood (Muscatine study), cardiovascular organogenesis and development, cardiac electrophysiology, and echocardiography. Dr. Clark left the Division in 1985 to take a position at Johns Hopkins.

The Pediatric Ambulatory Division has been headed by Dr. Edem Ekwo since 1975. Other Ambulatory faculty include Drs. Brenda Cruikshank (1970), Vera Loening (1976), Lois Dusdieker (1979), Jerold Woodhead (1979), and Jody Murph (1985). Research interests include the pharmacotherapy of asthma and otitis media, breast feeding, immunization against haemophilus influenza, management of chronic constipation, the epidemiology of infectious diseases in day care centers, and Pediatric Nurse Practitioner training.

The Division of Developmental Disabilities has undergone a major transformation since the institution of Public Law 94-142 in 1977. The University Hospital School has been reorganized from a long-term, boarding school facility to a short-term, diagnostic evaluation center for inpatients and outpatients. Dr. Alfred Healey succeeded Dr. Raymond Remboldt as chairman of the Division in 1977. New faculty joining the Division include Drs. Mark Wolraich (1976), David Schor (1980), James Blackman (1981), and Randall Alexander (1984). The Division provides comprehensive interdisciplinary services to disabled children with help from dentistry, education, physical therapy, nursing, nutrition, occupational therapy, psychology, recreation, social services, speech pathology and audiology and vocational education. Areas of research include interdisciplinary training in developmental disabilities, child abuse and high-risk infant followup.

The Division of Pediatric Neurology is headed by Dr. William Bell. As a clinician and teacher he is much admired. He has been involved in clinical research, especially the clinical and laboratory evaluation of central nervous system infections. Dr. Erique Chavez was a member of the Division from 1975 to 1979, and Dr. Barry Bergen from 1980 to 1982. Dr. James Bale joined the Division in 1982; His research interests involve cytomegalovirus infection and its effect on host defenses. Dr. Adel K. Affifi joined the Division in 1984. His research involves neural connectivity in brainstem nuclei and histochemical and electron microscope features of neuromyopathies. Dr. Victor Ionasescu holds a joint appointment in pediatric neurology and staffs the neuromuscular disease clinic.

The Division of Pediatric Psychology was joined by Drs. Lynn Richman and Dennis Harper in 1974. Subsequently, Dr. Clarissa Holmes (1979), Scott Lindgren (1980), and David Wacker (1982) have become Division members. Areas of research interest include learning disabilities, neurodevelopmental screening, hyperkinetic children, psychosomatic disorders, neuropsychological functioning in diabetes mellitus, and patient-family dynamics in oncology patients.

Dr. Donald Mock became a member of the Division of Gastroenterology in 1985. His research interests are biotin metabolism and growth retardation in hereditary fructose intolerance. Dr. Younoszai's area of research is the growth and functional development of the gastrointestinal tract. The Division's clinical practice includes such procedures as gastrointestinal endoscopy, percutaneous liver biopsy, esophageal manometry and pH measurement, and hydrogen breath tests.

The Division of Biochemistry is headed by Dr. Lewis Stegink and Dr. Lloyd Filer holds a secondary appointment in the Division. In addition to performing laboratory amino acid anaysis for clinical services in the hospital, the Division has several research interests. These include parenteral nutrition, neurotoxic effects of dicarboxylic amino acids (i.e., aspartame), essential amino acid requirements with parenteral nutrition, new energy sources for IV nutrition in infants, and the metabolism of food additives. Some projects have involved collaboration with the Departments of Internal Medicine, Obstetrics, Surgery and Neuroanatomy.

Dr. Robert Roberts heads the Division of Clinical Pharmacology and

Toxicology with Drs. Weinberger, Ahrens, Weismann and Ekwo holding secondary appointments. The Division gives a formal course in clinical toxicology to pediatric residents and offers an elective in pediatric pharmacology. A book by Dr. Roberts, entitled *Drug Therapy in Infants,* was published in 1984 and represents a major contribution to the field of pediatric pharmacology.

The Division of Nutrition is headed by Dr. Samuel Fomon with additional members being Drs. Zeigler, Filer, and Rebouche (1984). The Division has a national and international reputation of excellence in the field of infant nutrition. Dr. Fomon's text *Infant Nutrition* is an authoritative work in the field. After relinquishing responsibility for patients with renal disease, Dr. Fomon's nutritional studies greatly expanded and came to involve a large number of infants living in the community. Until 1980 his teaching efforts in nutrition were directed largely toward post-doctoral training and continuing education, the latter consisting of a week-long intensive course in Pediatric Nutrition presented 45 times between 1968 and 1986. Enrollment at these courses has generally ranged from 80 to 100 persons, including dietitians and physicians from all parts of the United States and from a number of other countries. In 1980 Dr. Fomon became Director of the University of Iowa Program in Human Nutrition, a Ph.D.-degree program. Research interests of the Division of Nutrition have included dietary composition, food intake and growth, protein requirements of normal infants, iron absorption in infancy, carnitine requirements of normal infants, carnitine biosynthesis and metabolism, and nutritional supplements for the preterm infant fed human milk.

Dr. Fomon has served on several review panels of the National Institutes of Health and has consulted for a number of governmental agencies. His contributions in research and teaching have been recognized by a number of honors and awards: the Borden Award of the American Academy of Pediatrics; the Rosen von Rosenstein Medal of the Swedish Pediatric Society; a Doctor Honora Causa degree from the Catholic University, Cordoba, Argentina; the F. Cuenca Villoro Award, Zaragoza, Spain; the McCollum Award of the American Society for Clinical Nutrition; and honorary membership in the American Dietetic Association. He has served as President of the Midwest Society for Pediatric Research, as President of the American Society for Clinical Nutrition, and as Vice-president of the 12th International Congress of Nutrition.

The substantial enlargement of the pediatric faculty that has occurred since Dr. Smith's arrival has allowed more time for faculty research and resident teaching by decreasing somewhat the clinical responsibilities of the faculty. The Department has been reorganized administratively with the addition of more middle-management personnel. Research grants in the Pediatric Department totaled just under $6 million in 1986. This figure has remained stable despite cutbacks in available research monies. The development of ongoing, well-supported research has allowed the Department to grow.

PHYSICAL PLANT

The Pediatric Department has acquired practically all new facilities in the last ten years. The Department's first neonatal ICU opened on 4 West in 1975 with 12 beds. In 1981 the newly remodeled 4 West Intermediate Care Nursery opened; this was followed later the same year by the opening of the Pediatric Intensive Care Unit on the fifth floor of the Roy Carver Pavilion. In 1982 a new 11-bed Neonatal ICU opened and the Newborn Nursery was remodeled. The latest addition to the physical plant took place in late 1982 with the opening of the John Colloton Pavillion. This facility houses the new Pediatric Clinic, Infant (2JCW) and Bronchopulmonary Dysplasia (2JCE) Wards and Intermediate Intensive Care Unit on the second floor, and the Adolescent (3JCW) and Toddler (3JCE) Wards on the third floor.

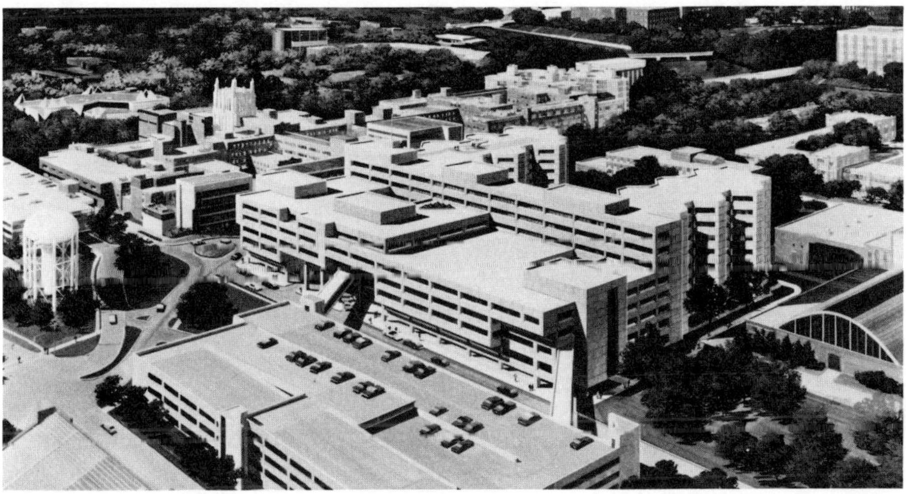

Architect's drawing of completed University Hospital with John Colloton Pavillion in the foreground.

RESIDENCY PROGRAM

The Pediatric Residency program has increased from seven residents per year to twelve residents in each level of training since 1973. In addition to the residency program, many of the pediatric subspecialties offer fellowship programs. In 1986 there were 20 Fellows in training in Pediatrics. The substantial growth of the Department in the areas of faculty, research, and clinical services has contributed to the building of a respected training program.

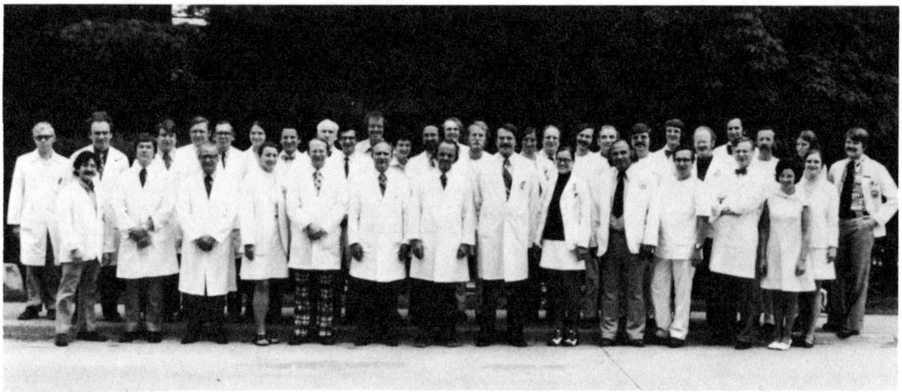

Pediatric faculty and house staff, 1973–74. *Front row:* L. Resnick, D. Harper, L. J. Filer, A. Kowal-Vern, R. Roberts, A. Healy, G. Baker, F. Smith, V. Visser, O. Ghazzawi, J. Binder, R. Lauer, B. Cruikshank, K. Mauer. *Second row:* J. Robillard, J. Stehbens, L. Richman, N. Karagan. J. Taylor, M. Waziri, S. Fomon, H. Zellweger, S. Kripke, B. Bartger, J. McDonnell, C. Johnson, C. Hayes, D. Weismann, G. McGuinness, C. T. Kisker, R. Sturdevant, V. Ionasescu, L. Mahoney, K. Anderson, P. Wallace, R. Schieken, R. Katnik, S. Mueller, J. Ashworth.

DEPARTMENT IN TRANSITION

Dr. Smith announced his plans to step down as Department Head in late 1984, and the search for his successor began. He will remain on the pediatric faculty and become involved in research in pediatric education. A scientific symposium honoring Dr. Smith's 13 years as Professor and Head of Pediatrics was held January 25, 1986. In February, 1986, he began a six-month sabattical to initiate his research and Dr. Robert Roberts served as acting Department Head. His many accomplishments and contributions to the Department of Pediatrics, pediatric education, and the health care of children in Iowa will long be remembered.

In July, 1986, Frank H. Morriss, Jr., M.D., was named Professor and Head of the Department of Pediatrics, effective January 1, 1987. Dr. Morriss had been Professor of Pediatrics, Obstetrics, and Gynecology, and Reproductive Sciences and Vice-chairman for Research and Development in the Department of Pediatrics at the University of Texas in Houston, having joined that faculty in 1973.

He received a bachelor's degree from the University of Virginia, where he was a Dupont Regional Scholar for four years, and an M.D. from Duke University Medical School. He completed internships in pathology and pediatrics and a pediatric residency at Duke before serving two years as a pediatrician at the Main Navy Dispensary in Washington, D.C. He returned to Duke for a one-year fellowship in neonatology before becoming a research fellow in perinatal medicine at the University of Colorado Medical Center, Denver.

Dr. Morriss was also a consultant in neonatology and pediatrics at several Houston hospitals and the M. D. Anderson Hospital and Tumor Institute and served as co-director of newborn service at Hermann Hospital.

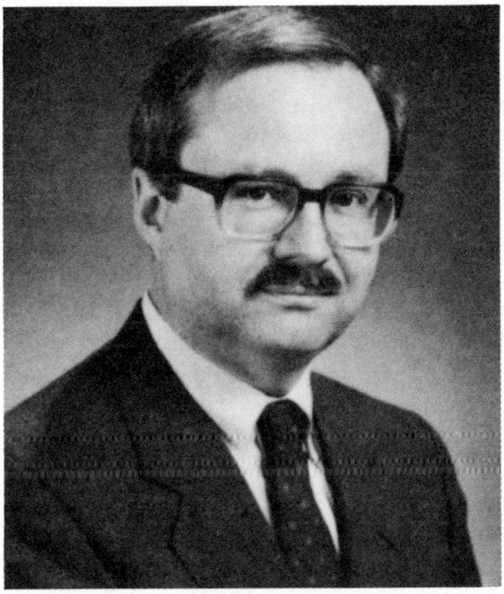

Frank Morriss, Jr., M.D.

Program of topics presented at the scientific symposium presented Saturday, January 25, 1986 to honor Fred G. Smith, Jr., M.D.:

1 STABLE ISOTOPE STUDIES OF ZINC METABOLISM IN INFANTS
E. Ziegler, Division of Nutrition

2 AMINOACID TURNOVER IN DIABETES MELLITIS
E. Tsalikian, Division of Endocrinology

3 BETA-ADRENERGIC AGONISM IN NEWBORN VENTRICULAR MYOCYTES
W. J. Marvin, Division of Cardiology

4 PHARMOCOKINETICS AND DYNAMICS OF INHALED BETA AGONISTS BY AIRWAY RESPONSIVENESS
R. C. Ahrens, Division of Allergy/Pulmonary

5 THE MAJOR ANTIGENS OF THE NEW CHICKEN POX VACCINE
C. F. Grose, Division of Infectious Disease

6 DEVELOPMENTAL NEPHROLOGY: THE FRED SMITH YEARS
J. Robillard, Division of Nephrology

7 MURINE CYTOMEGALOVIRUS GENOMIC MATERIAL IN BONE MARROW CELLS
J. F. Bale, Jr., Division of Neurology

8 LINKED GENES ON HUMAN CHROMOSOME—4
J. C. Murray, Division of Genetics

9 THE MECHANISM OF GROWTH RETARDATION IN HEREDITARY FRUCTOSE INTOLERANCE
D. M. Mock, Division of Gastroenterology

10 OXYGEN INDUCED LUNG INJURY
R. J. Roberts, Division of Clinical Pharmacology

11 EFFECTS OF HEAT SHIELDS ON THERMAL BALANCE OF RADIANTLY WARMED PREMATURE INFANTS
E. F. Bell, Division of Neonatology

12 FETAL DEVELOPMENT OF BLOOD COAGULATION
C. T. Kisker, Division of Hematology and Oncology

13 RELATIONSHIP OF PERINATAL FACTORS TO DEVELOPMENTAL OUTCOMES IN HIGH RISK INFANTS
J. A. Blackman, Division of Developmental Disabilities

14 LABORATORY TESTS OF RITALIN EFFECTS ON CLASSROOM ATTENTION AND BEHAVIOR
C. S. Holmes, Division of Psychology and B. M. Cruikshank, Division of Ambulatory Pediatrics

DEVELOPMENTAL NEPHROLOGY: THE FRED SMITH YEARS

Dr. Jean Robillard

Presented at the Scientific Symposium honoring Dr. Smith
January 25, 1986

Recent developments have added significantly to the body of knowledge required for the diagnosis and management of renal diseases in children. As a result, nephrology has emerged as a major subspecialty of pediatrics with many differences from its counterpart in internal medicine. One of the scientists who has contributed the most to the emergence of nephrology as a major discipline in pediatrics is Fred Smith.

Fred's career in academic medicine evolved over a period of about 25 years. It started in 1960, when he became an Assistant Professor of Pediatrics at UCLA Harbor General Hospital. In 1964 Fred moved to the UCLA Westwood Campus, where he stayed until 1973, at which time he moved to Iowa to become the Head of our Department.

At the beginning of his career, Fred developed an important interest in the study of the immunological mechanism involved in glomerulonephritis. His interests in that area were probably fostered by his year of fellowship in Minneapolis under the supervision of Dr. Robert Vernier and Dr. Robert Good. Also, looking at Dr. Smith's publications one will find a large number of manuscripts dealing with immune mechanisms controlling glomerular injury.

During the same period, Dr. Smith was also interested in endocrinology. In collaboration with Dr. F. Frasier at UCLA, he studied factors involved in growth retardation in children. However, his major contribution in the field of endocrinology has been his work on the development of the parathyroid function during fetal maturation. In a first series of papers, Dr. Smith studied the possible role of parathyroid hormone (PTH) in explaining the elevated phosphate observed in human neonates and immature animals. In a first study, he demonstrated that the decrease in fetal plasma calcium following infusion of EDTA was associated with an important increase in fetal plasma PTH. During the same period, he was able to demonstrate that there was a marked rise in urinary phosphate excretion associated with a rise in fetal plasma PTH. Taken together, these results suggested that the fetal PTH is responsive to alteration in fetal plasma calcium concentration and that the decreased ability of the fetal kidney to secrete phosphate may be due to low levels of PTH at birth.

In order to demonstrate that the rise in urinary phosphate excretion during induced hypocalcemia was directly dependent on a rise in PTH and not secondary to the hypocalcemia itself, Dr. Smith designed another study in which he evaluated the fetal renal response to PTH. This study, done in sheep, which was published in the *Journal of Applied Physiology* in 1969, demonstrated very clearly that infusion of parathyroid extract produced an increase in urinary phosphate excretion. This study demonstrated for the first time that a relative parathyroid insufficiency may be a major factor producing persistent high plasma phosphate concentration and low urinary phosphate excretion in immature animals and human newborns.

It is interesting to observe that, while Dr. Smith was still very productive in the endocrinology arena, he had already established himself as a pioneer in developmental nephrology. He foresaw as early as the late 1960s the survival of premature infants weighing less than 1 kilogram and anticipated the importance fluid and electrolyte metabolism would play in their care. Working with Pauline Alexander in London, he developed an animal model to study the maturation of renal function in premature animals and in so doing was the first investigator to study fetal renal function systematically. First Dr. Smith worked to develop an acute fetal preparation. Gross aspects of renal function were established in fetal monkeys and sheep. He demonstrated that the glomerular filtration rate was in the range of 1 ml/min/kg of body weight in fetal animals and that the urine osmolality was less and 300 milliosmol/kg of water.

Probably Dr. Smith's major accomplishment in developmental nephrology has been his work on the renin-angiotensin system. In 1974 he published a paper entitled "The renin-angiotensin system in the fetal lamb" in *Pediatric Research.* This work represents a landmark in his career for many reasons. First, it was his last project completed at UCLA before becoming Department Head at the University of Iowa. Second, this paper now represents a cornerstone in our knowledge of the ontogeny of the renin-angiotensin system. For the first time, an investigator was able to show that the renin-angiotensin system was functional during fetal life. Moreover, it was demonstrated that plasma renin activity levels were higher in fetal animals than in the mothers. This study has been cited more than 100 times already in the literature and has been at the origin of a series of studies looking at factors controlling renin secretion during development.

When Dr. Smith moved to Iowa City in 1973 he decided that physiological studies in fetal animals should be done without the stress of surgery or anesthesia. He also developed a chronic fetal model to study the development of renal function during gestation. Using that model, which is still extensively used in fetal nephrology, he and his collaborators were able to study the maturation of the glomerular filtration rate, factors modulating sodium metabolism, water metabolism and acid base balance. More recently, the effect of hypoxemia and hemorrhage on the maturation of the fetal function have also been investigated.

Because of his work in research and his remarkable interest in pediatric nephrology, Dr. Smith was elected President of the American Pediatric Nephrology Society in 1977. Since that time, he has continued to be very active in the field of pediatric nephrology, and his work will continue to be considered landmarks in the field.

DR. SMITH'S FAREWELL

Presented by Dr. Herman Hein
January 25, 1986

This is a very special day for all who have been associated with Fred Smith. In spite of all that has been said and will be said, we recognize that we cannot adequately thank him for his devotion to us and to Iowa's children.

Fred's legacy is extensive. This morning we gathered to pay tribute to the new vistas in pediatric research that Fred has fostered over the past twelve years. Also, he is loved and respected as the consummate teacher. Students, house staff, and faculty have been enriched by his devotion to pediatric education. Currently, over one-third of all practicing pediatricians in Iowa were trained by Fred.

Fred is also revered as a skilled and caring physician. Not only has he taught patient care, but also has personally provided care to a large number of very sick children in spite of his overwhelming time commitment as Department Head.

There are many other examples that could be offered to illustrate Fred's impact on the Department, the College of Medicine, and the University. However, his influence has not been limited to the University of Iowa. Rather, the entire state has benefited from his skill and devotion.

Since 1973, a number of programs have been developed which have had a salutary effect on all of Iowa's children. Time does not permit a thorough recounting of all these efforts, but I will share several highlights with you.

I am sure that many of you are aware of John MacQueen's work to provide services for Iowa's children with chronic problems. His State Services for Crippled Children Program, now known as Child Health Specialty Clinics, has offered specialized services to needy children close to their homes. During the past twelve years, these programs have expanded to include specialized regional clinics, staffed by interdisciplinary personnel, which are designed to evaluate children with developmental problems and to offer treatment programs for the children as close to their homes as possible. In 1985, 6,413 children received specialized diagnostic and treatment services during visits to CHSC mobile and regional clinics. The mobile and regional clinics not only increase the availability of specialized health services to children, but also result in considerable cost savings to their families.

Jim Hanson and the Division of Medical Genetics, following the pioneering work of Hans Zellweger, have been instrumental in developing a statewide network of genetic evaluation and counseling services as well as other essential services. Working with Drs. John Goodrich and Ted Scurletis of the Iowa State Health Department, the Statewide Newborn Genetics and Metabolic Screening Program was renovated and currently services some 45,000 Iowa newborns yearly. The Division of Medical Genetics has contributed to the development of a statewide maternal alpha-fetoprotein screening program as well. A system of sixteen regional genetic counseling clinic sites has been established and currently serves 800–1,000 Iowa families at sites away from University Hospitals. In addition, the Regional program staff conducts 200–250 educational programs annually throughout the state. In 1970, the Division was seeing some 200 families per year at University Hospitals. Now, it provides clinical, diagnostic, and counseling services for genetic disorders, birth defects, and neuromuscular conditions to some 900 families yearly, as well as providing nearly 1,500 cytogenetic analyses annually. A statewide birth defects registry and a new project to provide information on teratogens to Iowa families and physicians have also recently been developed.

Dr. Tom Kisker and other members of the Hematology Division have fostered the development of care programs for children with cancer and hemophilia. These programs are designed so that the children can receive as much care near their homes as posssible. The Childhood Cancer Diagnostic and Treatment Network originated in 1977. At the present time, more than 150 children are actively receiving on-going care in their local communities from more than 110 different local practitioners. This program allows State of the Art care to pediatric oncology patients regardless of their residence, and allows patients and their families to maintain their local support during very difficult and stressful treatment. Furthermore, the program results in considerable savings in travel cost and time lost in gainful employment by parents.

The Rural Comprehensive Care Program for Hemophilia began in 1978. Initially there were 25 patients; currently over 260 hemophilia patients receive comprehensive care through the University of Iowa center. Because of the center, absenteeism from school as a result of problems associated with the bleeding disorder has been significantly reduced, and unemployment rates of adult hemophilia patients has been markedly reduced for the past two years.

Since 1973, a statewide system of regional perinatal health care has been developed for Iowa. This system includes 11 regional perinatal centers in addition to the University of Iowa. This care network allows pregnant women and newborn babies to receive services as close to their home as possible. The University of Iowa provides backup services for all of the regional perinatal centers. The year prior to Fred's coming to Iowa, nearly 15 of every 1,000 babies born died before they reached 28 days of age. Currently, this figure has been reduced to approximately 5 per 1,000. In simple human terms, this means that approximately 460 fewer babies die each year prior to reaching one month of age.

Also, the special needs of the infants that require neonatal intensive care have been recognized and a statewide system of high-risk infant follow-up has been developed over the past ten years. This system, a cooperative venture of the Statewide Perinatal Care Program, the Child Health Specialty Clinics, the Divisions of Developmental Disabilities and Neonatology, and Iowa community hospitals, ensures that neonates who are at high-risk for medical and development problems receive diagnostic services on a regular basis. Problems are identified as soon as possible and appropriate remedial action taken. I believe Fred is particularly pleased that the programs interrelate to best meet the needs of Iowa's children. As noted, the Followup Program is a joint venture using public and private resources to serve children. The hemophilia program and Child Health Specialty Clinics are developing a cooperative program to ensure appropriate treatment for their patients at the local level. Also, genetic counseling for hemophilia families is provided by Dr. Hanson's Statewide Network.

Knowing Fred as well as I do, I am sure that he is protesting that these programs are not his work, but rather the work of others. The truth of the matter is that Fred helped to cultivate the environment and the individuals which allowed the various programs to spawn and then he supported their growth.

Fred has never been one to seek applause and frequently goes out of his way to ensure that others receive credit for their efforts. Fred, all of us working with the programs for Iowa's children recognize your many contributions and unfailing support for these programs. We thank you for ourselves, and most importantly, for the children of Iowa.

A HISTORY OF UNIVERSITY HOSPITAL SCHOOL

University Hospital School (UHS) began serving disabled children on October 13, 1948, through a small legislative appropriation that was used to initiate a program in the basement of Westlawn on the University of Iowa campus. The appropriation was the result of a provision enacted by the 52nd General Assembly of the State of Iowa calling for the creation of a state hospital school for severely handicapped children. All enrollees were severely physically handicapped, but capable of profiting from a specially designed educational program. The initial enrollment of eight children expanded to 20 by the end of the first year.

In January of 1954 the program moved into a new building, known as University Hospital School for Severely Handicapped Children, located to the west of University Hospitals. The new facility included accommodations for 60 residential students, an industrial arts shop, gymnasium, food service facility, play equipment, wading pool, and recreational rooms.

Admission to UHS was usually recommended for children who, because of their severe physical disability, could not reach their optimum level of academic achievement in their schools, but who showed promise of being able to do so after a period of residence. Typically, such children attended UHS during the usual nine-month school term for two or three years. Other children who were disabled and attending local schools were frequently admitted for two months during summers to enhance their local school performance. During their admission at UHS, children received interdisciplinary service from professionals in the fields of medicine, dental and nursing care, communication skills, physical and occupational therapy, special education, physical education, industrial arts, homemaking, music, and child development.

The UHS building and program expanded in 1964 to include The Pine School and Child Development Clinic. A new south wing was constructed for these programs with funds provided by Public Law 88-164 (Construction of Mental Retardation Facilities), which allocated monies to assist in programming for children with intellectual handicaps.

The Child Development Clinic provided outpatient diagnostic guidance services for children with problems suggestive of mental retardation or relating to poor school performance and psychological problems associated with medical conditions. Pine School was a day-school for 90 Iowa City area children, ages 3 to 17, who functioned in the trainable and educable ranges of mental retardation. As a cooperative venture between the Iowa City School District and the Division of Special Education, College of Education, the Pine School provided a training site for students preparing for a career in special education.

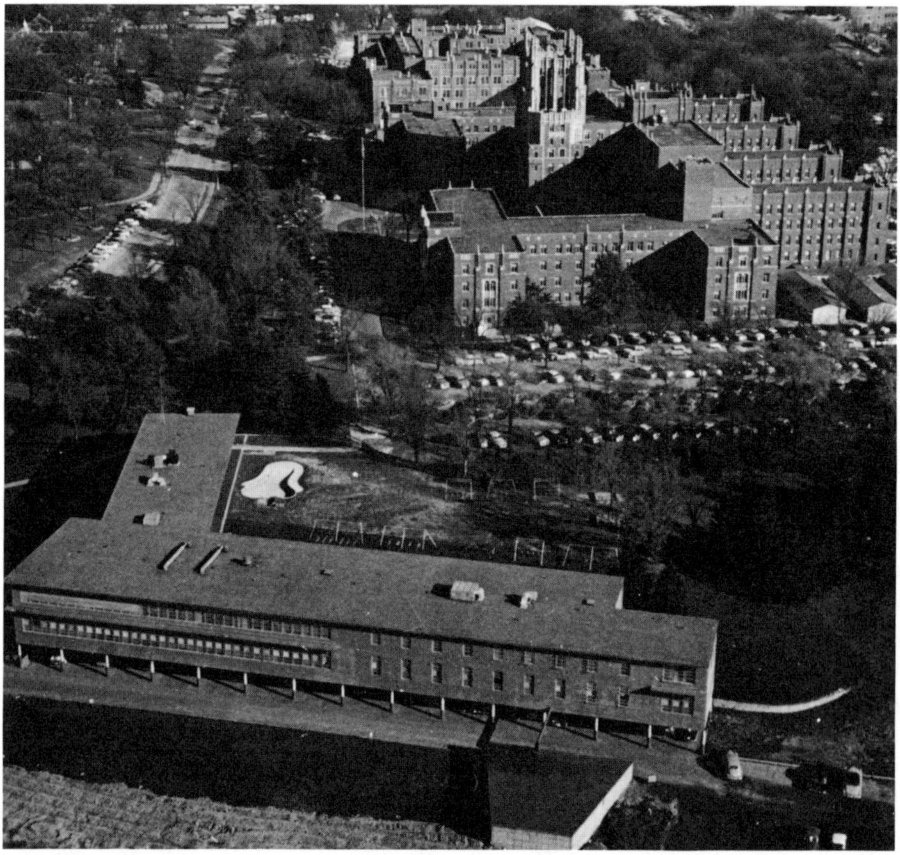

University Hospital School for Severely Handicapped Children at the time of its opening in 1954. The University Hospital and Medical Laboratories are seen in the background.

In 1972 UHS accepted a new role as a University Affiliated Facility (UAF). UAFs were the nation's first major federally sponsored initiative to provide interdisciplinary training, exemplary service, and research to assist persons with mental retardation, cerebral palsy, and epilepsy. This definition was later expanded to include other disablilities. As a UAF, the UHS extended its program by providing interdisciplinary training, dissemination of information, technical assistance, and applied research for personnel who work with disabled children and adults.

The 1970s also brought about passage of new public laws that resulted in important changes affecting the lives of disabled persons and the types and methods of services provided for them. The adoption in 1975 of "The Education for All Handicapped Children Act" (Public Law 94-142), stating that all children have a right to a free and appropriate public education in their home communities, brought about the creation of community-based education, care, and treatment programs for individuals with severe disabilities. Similar state legislation (Senate file 1163) called for the creation of Area Education Agencies to support the needs of children requiring special education and a method for financing programs and services.

As children and young adults previously served at UHS were integrated into community-based programs, UHS placed increased emphasis on outclinic and outreach services in support of these community programs. Inpatient services were modified to help patients achieve goals that could be accomplished within a relatively short admission period. Pine School was also discontinued as its enrollees were mainstreamed into public schools.

The UHS became affiliated in 1977 with the University of Iowa Hospitals and Clinics as the Division of Developmental Disabilities in the Department of Pediatrics. That change gave Division patients direct access to specialized medical care as a part of their comprehensive interdisciplinary services.

Today the Division of Developmental Disabilities serves as the focus for a wide variety of patient services, training programs, and research endeavors relative to children and young adults with developmental disabilities. Patient services are especially designed to address the needs of patients with complex and interrelated physical, intellectual, learning and/or adjustment problems. The following professional disciplines provide evaluations, either routinely or upon consultation as needed: audiology, dentistry, education, medicine, nursing, nutrition, occupational therapy, physical therapy, psychology, recreation, social services, and speech and language pathology.

Most patients of the Division are seen in one of the five outclinics that provide diagnostic evaluations and/or management and follow-up services: The Infant and Young Child Clinic, for suspected of confirmed developmental disabilities in children, ages birth to three and over; Child Development Clinic, for children with poor school performance, learning disabilities, hyperactivity, mild behavior disorders and/or problems associated with suspected child abuse and/or neglect; Myelodysplasia Clinic, for spinal cord disorders; and The Metabolic Management Clinic, for metabolic disorders that require long-term monitoring and special care.

Outpatient evaluations routinely lead to recommendations of treatment plans being formulated for patients in consultation with local physicians, schools, and other providers of service. These plans may include continued follow-up on an outpatient basis and/or admission to the inpatient unit.

Admission to the inpatient unit is often recommended to assist a patient in acheiving a specific short-term goal. Examples of reasons for admissions may include implementing a feeding program, intensive training with ambulation devices, medication adjustments and/or intensive evaluation of a child's disabilities. Other reasons may involve determining what special equipment will increase a patient's independence. Modified wheelchairs for positioning to enhance function and to offset skin and skeletal problems are prescribed, modified and/ or constructed within the inpatient unit.

These interdisciplinary services include ongoing collaborative programs with a variety of clinical departments and other divisions of the Department of Pediatrics. For example: patients of the Myelodysplasia Clinic are routinely followed in cooperation with the Departments of Urology and Orthopedics; many patients are seen in the Child and Young Adult Clinic with the Department of Orthopedics; many are seen in the Infant and Young Child Clinic as a result of referrals from the Division of Neonatology; special inpatient care is provided for selected patients of the Division of Allergy/Pulmonary Diseases; and the Metabolic Management Clinic functions in collaboration with the Division of Medical Genetics.

The Division's training and research programs are also interdisciplinary. A total of 22 staff members hold faculty appointments in Pediatrics or other University departments. Specific training programs are routinely ongoing for students and clinical practitioners from all of the Division's disciplines. Therefore, the broad interdisciplinary base of service, training and research permits the Division of Developmental Disabilities to keep pace in fulfilling its mission to assist in reducing health and functional barriers to education, employment, and the enjoyment of life that confront children and young adults with developmental disabilities and chronic health impairments.

A HISTORY OF THE DIVISION OF MEDICAL GENETICS

During the first half of the 20th century, a growing body of clinical information made it increasingly clear that a significant number of human health problems had genetic bases. The work of Archibald Garrod, the rediscovery of Mendel's laws, and many other contributions advanced the study of human genetic disorders; but the basic chemical structure of the genetic material of man was not identified until the middle 1950s, by Watson and Crick. Likewise, it was only in the 1950s that techniques were developed which would allow the correct number of human chromosomes, 46, to be identified. Then, in 1959, Down's syndrome became the first identified chromosomal disorder of man, and with these developments was ushered in an explosive era of growth in the knowledge of human genetics.

Prior to the 1960s, then, there were no genetics clinics, chromosome labs, prenatal diagnosis programs, or many of the other facilties and programs which we associate with clinical genetics today. Indeed, the term "genetic counseling" had not yet been coined by Sheldon Reed; and, for most physicians, genetics was an obscure subject of little practical value.

At this critical juncture, a central figure in the development of clinical genetics at the University of Iowa appeared. Dr. Hans Zellweger, a Swiss pediatrician and protégé of the renowned Guido Fanconi and later a co-worker with Dr. Albert Schweitzer in Lambarene, French Equatorial Africa, was persuaded by Dean Norman Nelson of the University of Iowa College of Medicine to leave his post as Chairman of the Department of Pediatrics at the American University in Beirut, Lebanon, to spend a sabbatical year (1957–58) in the Department of Pediatrics in Iowa City.

Dr. Zellweger had long been interested in neurological and neuromuscular disorders in childhood as well as other birth defect conditions. While he intended to continue his studies in this area during his sabbatical year at Iowa, his plans were disrupted at the outset by the precipitous departure of Dr. Charles May, Professor and Head of the Department of Pediatrics. As a consequence, Zellweger's attentions were focused in a somewhat different area; and in that sabbatical year he made his first contribution to genetics at Iowa. A dietary approach to the prevention of mental retardation from phenylketonuria had been

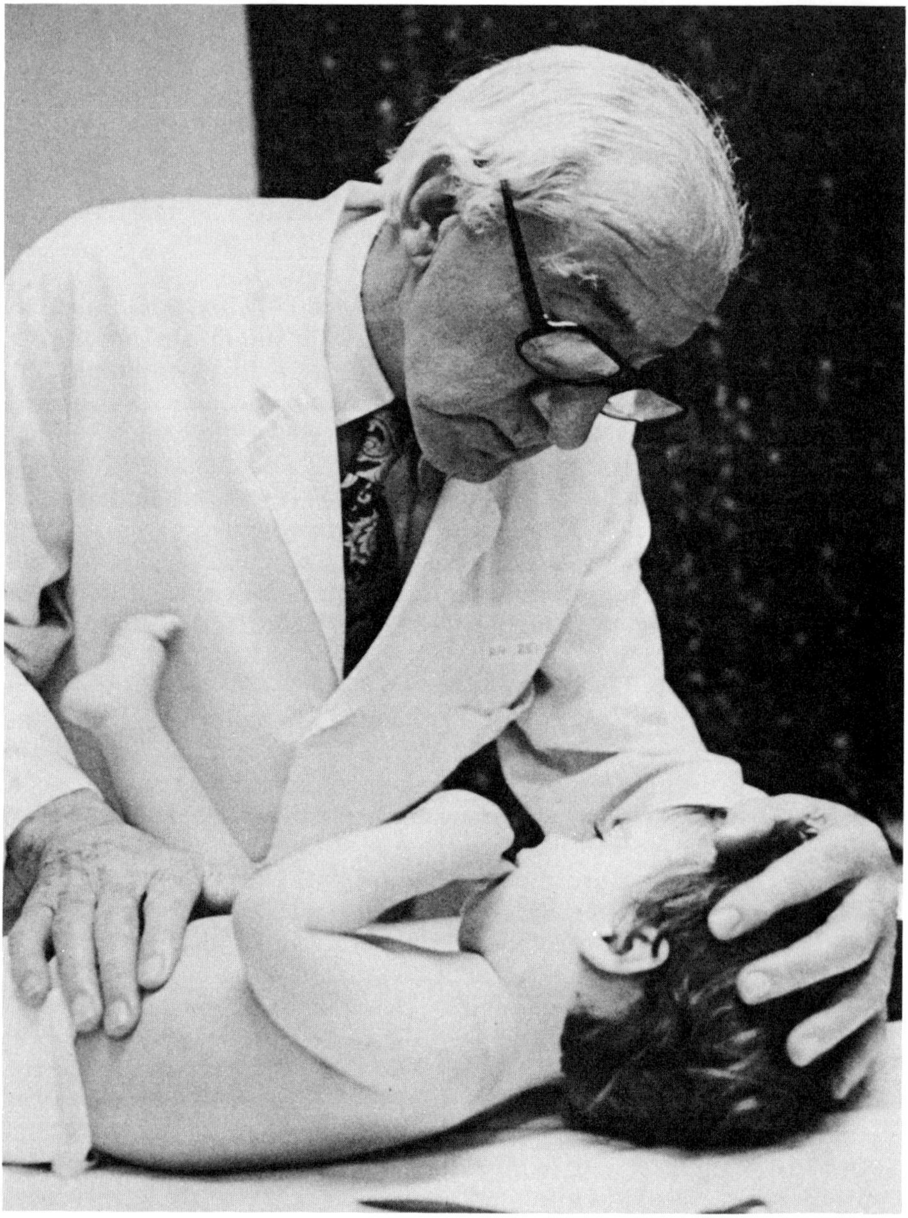

Hans Zellweger, M.D.

proposed. This attracted the interest of Zellweger and a young pediatrician, Dorothy Ehmke, who was later to join Dr. Jacqueline Noonan in the Division of Pediatric Cardiology. Dr. Ehmke had trained previously as a dietitian, and these skills were of great value in her collaboration with Dr. Zellweger in the formation of the Department's first PKU clinic. This clinic was to form the foundation for what ultimately has developed into a statewide program for screening and treatment of children with a number of genetic/metabolic conditions.

In 1958, Dr. Zellweger left Iowa City briefly to conclude his tenure at Beirut before returning permanently to the University of Iowa as Professor of Pediatrics in 1959. This was to prove a momentous year, which began with Zellweger helping to establish a true interdisciplinary spina bifida clinic in the Department of Pediatrics with a grant from the National Foundation of the March of Dimes, which had recently switched its focus from polio to birth defects. Unfortunately, however, for the spina bifida clinic, in 1959 Herome Lejeune announced the identification of an extra small acrocentic chromosome in patients with Down's syndrome. This work and that of other human cytogeneticists, such as Patricia Jacobs and Arthur Robinson, caught the attention of Zellweger, who approached his fellow Swiss countryman, Emil Witschi, Ph.D., Professor of Zoology in the Graduate College. Witschi had been interested in studying chromosomes in mice for some time and agreed to help Zellweger establish a human cytogenetics laboratory. In 1960 the two were successful in obtaining a $10,000 grant from the National Institutes of Health to start a facility, which became one of the first human cytogenetics laboratories in the United States. Working with Zellweger in this lab were a post-doctoral fellow from Zoology, Jun-bi Tu, and a young medical student, John Opitz, who was later to distinguish himself as a clinical geneticist at the University of Wisconsin and, subsequently, as editor of the *American Journal of Medical Genetics.*

During that first year, the laboratory studied both human and rodent chromosomes and a sound scientific basis for an important clinical service and research activity was thereby established. This laboratory now carries out over 1,600 analyses per year on patients with birth defect problems, families seeking prenatal diagnosis of congenital disorders and on patients with various forms of cancer.

In 1961 Zellweger started the first genetics clinic at the University of Iowa and offered a course on genetics to the medical students. However, over the next two years relatively few patients came to this clinic. Perplexed by this, Dr. Zellweger sought counsel from, among others, Dr. Elmer DeGowin of the Department of Internal Medicine, who advised him first to educate the faculty.

Dr. Zellweger subsequently obtained a $2,000 grant from the Dean of the College of Medicine, Dr. Robert Hardin, and in 1963 conducted a course in human genetics for the faculty of the College of Medicine. This course, which lasted eight evenings, included a number of illustious guests, including Dr. Victor McKusick of Johns Hopkins Hospital, Dr. James Neel of the University of Michigan, Dr. James Crow of the University of Wisconsin, and Dr. Elving Anderson of the University of

Minnesota, as well as others from the University of Iowa, especially Dr. Opitz. This course had a most salutary effect and the growth and ultimate success of the Genetics Clinic was thereby assured.

During the middle 1960s, Dr. Zellweger continued his interests in human cytogenetic disorders and birth defects and yet found time to return to an earlier love: neuromuscular disorders. He founded a clinic for children and adults with muscular dystophies and other neuromuscular conditions and contributed significantly to the delineation of many uncommon myopathic syndromes and metabolic disorders of muscle. He also continued his clinical studies of various birth defect problems through the Genetics Clinic and in 1963 encountered an infant with profound hypotonia, dysmorphic facial features and CNS, hepatic and renal abnormalities, which he correctly diagnosed as a unique disorder. This condition, now known as the cerebro-hepatorenal syndrome, or the Zellweger syndrome, has been recognized as the prototypic peroxisomal metabolic disorder. During this period, he also wrote extensively on the Prader-Willi syndrome and a variety of human chromosomal disorders. This truly represented a remarkable decade of achievement for a single pediatrician/clinical geneticist who was assisted by two or three laboratory technicians, a secretary, a clinic coordinator who doubled as an administrative assistant, and a scattering of medical students and other trainees.

In 1969 Dr. Zellweger was joined by Dr. Victor Ionasescu, a Rumanian neurologist whose interest in neuromuscular disorders and muscle biochemistry led to the development of a muscle research laboratory within the Division and soon thereafter the establishment, with the encouragement and assistance of Dr. John MacQueen, of one of the country's first neuromuscular field clinic programs.

In 1973 the Department of Pediatrics was reorganized under the leadership of a new Department Head, Dr. Fred Smith. With this process came the recognition of a separate Division of Medical Genetics with Dr. Zellweger as its Chairman. Over the next few years Zellweger, assisted by Jane Simpson, a nurse interested in genetic counseling, began to explore the possibility of providing genetic counseling clinics in other parts of Iowa. These efforts, substantially aided by the state director of Maternal and Child Health, Dr. Theodore Scurletis, and several local legislators, culminated in 1976 in the enactment by the Legislature of a statute empowering the Iowa Department of Health to establish a statewide Regional Genetic Consultation Service. This was the first step in the development of a statewide comprehensive program of genetics health care services. Zellweger was named Clinical Director of this program in 1976, and he served in that capacity until 1980.

In 1976, Dr. James Hanson joined the faculty of the Division. He had been a student research fellow with Zellweger while in medical school at the University of Iowa from 1965 through 1969. His appointment to the Division strengthened its emphasis on general clinical genetics, dysmorphology, and teratogenesis and also allowed Zellweger to concentrate on the development of the first pilot phase of the Regional Genetics Consultation Service in northeastern Iowa, all with the assistance of Mrs. Simpson and a second nurse, Elizabeth Thomson.

Also in 1976, Dr. Mary Waziri, a pediatrician with additional training in medical genetics under Dr. Zellweger, became an Associate in Pediatrics in the Division. Her interests in clinical aspects of genetic disorders associated with cancer and in the phakomatoses, including neurofibromatosis, has subsequently evolved into significant clinical research and service programs.

In 1977 Dr. Zellweger was appointed Professor Emeritus of Pediatrics at the University of Iowa and Dr. Hanson assumed the Chairmanship of the Division, with Dr. Ionasescu becoming responsible for the neuromuscular portion of the program. During the next two years, the dramatic success of the Regional Genetic Consultation Service led the Legislature to expand the program statewide and ushered in a period of explosive growth.

In 1978 Shivanand Patil, Ph.D., was appointed to the Division faculty as Director of the Cytogenetics Laboratory; and in 1979 William Rhead, M.D., Ph.D., and James Bartley, M.D., Ph.D., were added to the Division faculty not only to strengthen the Division's clinical faculty, but also to broaden its capabilities in the areas of biochemical and developmental genetics.

Concurrently with these developments, faculty members of the Division of Medical Genetics joined with faculty members in the College of Medicine and Graduate School departments to initiate an Inter-department Ph.D. Program in Genetics at the University and collaborated with the staff of the Birth Defects Institute of the Iowa State Department of Health in reorganizing the state's program for newborn metabolic and genetic screening. In addition, an extensive outreach educational program regarding genetics and health was developed which also had a significant impact on the knowledge and attitudes of Iowa physicians and health care providers and the general public regarding the utilization of genetic health care services. Furthermore, during this period, a post-doctoral, clinical, and research fellowship training program in medical genetics was established. This program has since been accredited by the American Board of Medical Genetics for training of physicians in clinical genetics and related areas.

In 1984 Dr. Jeffrey Murray joined the Division to head a laboratory research program in molecular genetics; and in 1985 Dr. Wilma Krause joined the Division as the new Director of the Metabolic Management Clinic. Krause and Murray also brought substantial additional clinical strength to the Division.

The year 1986 has seen a continuation of the development of new Divisional programs with the initiation of a statewide Birth Defects Registry program under the aegis of the Iowa Department of Health and the U.S. Centers for Disease Control, the establishment of a teratogen information service, the development of a statewide maternal serum alpha-fetoprotein testing program in conjunction with the Department of Obstetrics and Gynecology and the University Hygenic Laboratory, and new proposals for extended newborn screening, molecular testing, and environmental surveillance activities.

The Division now serves some 1600 to 1800 families yearly in its university and outreach clinic programs which are now held in 16 Iowa cities. It provides some 200 to 250 educational programs each year around the state to health professionals, educators, other professional groups, students and the general public. It supervises the clinical care and management of children with metabolic/genetic disorders and other birth defects throughout the state and provides a host of laboratory diagnostic services and research programs to the University Hospitals and to the people of Iowa. It offers training opportunities for medical students, students from other health professions, postdoctoral fellows, graduate students in genetics and many postgraduate continuing education programs. The Division of Medical Genetics at the University of Iowa serves as the coordination center for the Great Plains Genetics Service Network, an eight-state regional organization of clinical genetics, crippled children's, and maternal and child health programs.

APPENDIX A

Physicians completing postgraduate training in Pediatrics at the University of Iowa Hospitals and Clinics from 1915 to July 1986.

Name	*Dates*
Agha, Amad	1976–1978
Alejandrino, Lourdes	1956–1958
Al-Rashid, Rashid	1960–1961
Alsan, Nimet	1962–1963
Amick, Perry	1941–1943
Anderson, Kenneth	1972–1975
Anderson, Robert	1975–1978
Anneberg, Walter	1923–1924
Ansley, Steven	1971–1972
Ardinger, Holly	1983–1984
Ardinger, Robert	1983–1986
Ardon, Marjorie	1968–1970
Aronberg, Dixie	1972–1973
Ashworth, James	1973–1974
Azimi, Parvin	1964–1965
Baker, George	1962–1964
Baker, Mary Lee	1980–1983
Balanoff, Arnold	1968–1970
Barkow, Kathleen	1975–1978
Barter, Bruce	1972–1974
Bayne, Edward	1974–1977
Beal, Douglas	1980–1983
Beerends, Jerold	1974–1977
Berg, John	1950–1952
Berry, Paul	1981–1984
Binder, John	1973–1976
Bitar, John	1962–1963
Blau, Alice	1941–1944
Bleicher, Stacie	1979–1982
Block, Walter	1946–1947
Bonde, Denise	1983–1986
Bowen, R.	1924
Boysen, James	1951–1954
Brennan, John	1967–1968
Brown, William	1976–1979
Bryan, George	1956–1958
Burkeholder, James	1961–1963
Butterbrodt, Mark	1977–1980
Carney, Thomas	1959–1960
Cass, Kathleen	1977–1980
Chandramouli, B.	1966–1967
Chinnock, Robert	1947–1948
Comly, Hunter	1944–1946
Cook, David	1983–1986
Connell, Bernard	1979–1982
Cooney, Lawrence	1981–1984
Cooper, Jeffrey	1978–1981
Copeland, Linda	1981–1984
Cowan, Anthony	1962–1963
Cramblett, Henry	1956–1958
Cusminsky, Marcos	1960–1961
Cuthbertson, Gilbert	1983–1986
Daws, William	1976–1979
deGuzman, Ricardo	1957–1958
Dick, Mark	1933–1935
Dine, Mark	1951–1952
Dixon, David	1976–1979
dos Remedios, Leonardo	1948–1949
Dover, Arthur	1971–1972
Downing, John	1945–1947
Durnin, Robert	1960–1962
Dworet, Rochelle	1975–1977
Ebers, Douglas	1983–1986
Edwards, M. Thomas	1977–1980
Ehmke, Dorothy	1957–1959
Ekermeyer, Ernest	1933–1934
Eldredge, Eugene	1953–1955
Elzouki, Abdelaziz	1974–1976
Evans, Jonathon	1981–1984
Falkenstein, Dorothy	1938–1940
Feist, James	1974–1977
Finnegan, Jerald	1968–1969
Firestone, James	1980–1983

Fisher, Eileen 1981–1984
Fisk, Charlotte 1935–1936
Fletcher, Larry 1970–1972
Floyd, Mark 1918–1919
Foster, Morgan 1922–1923
Fountain, Martha Toy 1981–1984
Franzen, Keevin 1976–1979
Freeman, Mable 1926–1927
French, Merle 1919–1920
Frost, Loraine 1949–1950
Fruehling, Carolyn 1976–1979

Garbade, Francis 1931–1932
Gauchat, Robert 1952–1954
Geddie, Kenneth 1927–1928
Gerken, James K. 1921–1923
Ghazzawi, Omar 1973–1974
Gilbert, Joyce 1982–1985
Godfrey (Clawson), Charlene 1983–1986
Glass, Herbert 1950–1951
Goellner, Paul 1972–1973
Goerlich, Berthold 1954–1957
Goldberg, Marshall 1965–1967
Goldenberg, Leon 1949–1950
Gore, Bradley 1982–1983
Gould, Samuel 1953–1955
Graeve, Janet 1983–1986
Graven, Stanley 1958–1960
Green, Michael 1977–1978
Greenblatt, Jerald 1940–1942
Griffith, J. Edwin 1948–1950
Grino, Marie 1959–1961

Hackbarth, Stanley 1977–1980
Hacker, Mary 1969–1971
Haddad, Nadra 1959–1960
Halmi, Katherine 1966–1968
Hansen, James 1982–1985
Hare, James 1955–1957
Harner, Marvin 1968–1971
Harris, Dorris 1957–1959
Harris, James 1980–1983
Harrison, G. E. 1928–1930
Hawit, Raja 1966–1968
Hayek, J. M. 1926–1927
Healy, Alfred 1964–1966
Hein, Herman 1965–1966
Heitsman, Jay 1978–1981
Heller, Joseph 1962–1964
Henderson, R. W. 1921–1922
Hendrix, James 1975–1977
Henkin, J. H. 1915–1916
Henning, G. G. 1929–1931
Hippchen, Ray 1962–1964
Horning, Marguerite 1927–1929
Howard, William 1935–1936
Huff (Dennis), Denise 1963–1965
Huges, R. O. 1929–1930
Hughes, Vivian 1952–1953
Hunt, Mary Ann 1953–1954

Isom, John 1955–1956

Jackson, Robert 1934–1935
1936–1937
Jackson, William 1963–1965
Jaeger, Waltraud 1958–1959
Jain, P.S. 1919–1920
Jameson, W.B. 1927–1928
Jimenez, Daniel 1976–1979
Johnson, Lawrence 1974–1977
Joad, Jesse 1978–1981

Kahn, Joseph 1977–1980
Kantrow, Abraham 1935–1936
Karlsson, Maud 1970–1972
Katnik, Richard 1973–1975
Kayyali, M. Zafer 1969–1971
Kehoe, Joseph 1947–1949
Kemp, David 1975–1978
Kidd, William 1970–1972
Kiehl, Phyllis 1970–1971
King, James 1964–1966
Kittams, Brian 1978–1981
Klinsman, R. P. 1926–1927
Knorr, William 1974–1977
Knox, Joseph 1925–1926
Knudson, Lon 1978–1981
Kobayashi, Clifford 1946–1948

Koellner, Paul	1961–1963
Kousseff, Boris	1970–1971
Kowal Vern, Areta	1972–1974
Kuehn, Harold	1964–1966
Lababidi, Zuhdi	1967–1968
Lammer, Edward	1979–1982
Larew, Mary	1981–1983
Lascari, Andre	1962–1963
Laubscher, J. Howard	1944–1945
Lee, Keun	1968–1969
Levine, Stanley	1971–1974
Liedman, Jay	1976–1979
Lilian, Bernard	1934–1935
Lillie, Michele	1981–1984
Linder, Jean	1968–1969
Lintermans, John	1960–1962
Linton, Randall	1978–1981
Mackler, Bruce	1946–1947
MacQueen, John	1947–1949
Maguire, Grace	1974–1977
Mahoney, Larry	1973–1976
Manges, Boyd	1983–1986
Marsh, Richard	1977–1980
Marshall, Bruce	1948–1950
Marvin, William	1974–1975
Matelich, Craig	1982–1985
Matson, Steven	1983–1986
Mauer, Katharine	1973–1974
Mayfield, Steven	1980–1983
McArthur, James	1953–1955
McAveney, William	1967–1968
McBride, Robert	1923–1925
McCray, Paul	1981–1984
McCubbin, Michael	1977–1980
McDonnell, Jean	1968–1969
McGill, R. Michael	1982–1985
McGuinness, Gail	1972–1975
McIntosh, C. B.	1942–1943
McLeod, Mary	1936–1937
McMullen, Jane	1945–1946
Merida, Joaquin	1960–1961
Merrick, James	1976–1978
Meyer, Paul	1981–1984
Miller, Debra	1980–1983
Miller, Philip	1977–1981
Mirhij, Najwa	1974–1976
Mirkhani, Mahmood	1956–1957
Mischler, Elaine	1970–1971
Mitchell, Gertrude	1933–1934
Mitchell, Richard	1952–1953
Moffett, Hugh	1957–1960
Montana, Eduardo	1964–1965
Moon, Herbert	1917–1919
Mueller, Shirley	1971–1974
Mullick, Umesh	1965–1966
Murph, Jody	1979–1982
Naficy, Kiarash	1959–1961
Najjar, Samir	1957–1959
Nakamura, Kenneth	1979–1982
Nassif, Edward	1975–1978
Nassif, Sami	1957–1959
Nau, Bradley	1981–1984
Nau, Scott	1978–1981
Nelsen, Carl	1962–1963
Niccum, Warren	1951–1953
Nordin, James	1974–1977
Norins, Nan	1983–1986
Normanly, Jerrod	1968–1969
Nye, Lillian	1920–1921
Odell, James	1953–1955
Olgac, Sezai	1961–1962
Opitz, John	1959–1961
Osborn, Sandra	1970–1972
Ovacik, Ekrem	1960–1962
Owen, George	1956–1958
Pabst, Mark	1963–1965
Park, Keun Lee	1968–1969
Paschal, G. A.	1929–1931
Patton, Charles	1953–1955
Payne, Catherine	1974–1975
Pearson, Nancy	1976–1979
Peitso, Marilyn	1979–1982
Perdue, Judith	1981–1985
Perozzi, Thelma	1934–1935
Pertuz, Marco	1961–1962

Peterson, Harold	1932–1933
Piercy, Kenneth	1931–1932
Polage, David	1966–1969
Porter, Gerald	1959–1961
Potter, Jacob	1927–1929
Rames, Linda	1965–1967
Rao, P. T.	1951–1952
Rate, Peggy	1975–1977
Remboldt, Raymond	1946–1947
Resnick, Lewis	1973–1974
Reuben, Ronald	1947–1948
Riegle, Elaine	1967–1970
Rigas, Constantine	1970–1971
Ringle, Glenn	1984–1985
Roberts, B. W.	1925–1926
Roberts, Justus	1935–1936
Roberts, Robert	1970–1973
Rodemyer, Carole	1979–1982
Rosenberger, Thomas	1970–1973
Rothenberg, Lionel	1948–1949
Rozeboom, Paul	1967–1969
Russell, James	1920–1922
Salameh, Kamal	1964–1967
Scheinman, Jonathan	1967–1968
Schneider, Hansjorg	1966–1968
Schumann, Ellen	1981–1984
Schumacher, Beverly	1955–1958
Sell, Matthew	1980–1983
Shaddy, Robert	1980–1983
Shanaah, Younis	1970–1972
Sharpe, Larry	1971–1973
Shaw, Robert	1975–1978
Shirley, Hale	1927–1930
Simpson, Frederic	1941
Singer, J. E.	1937–1938
Sinning, John	1960–1961
Sinno, Anwar	1963–1965
Smith, Charles	1966–1969
Smythe, Arnold	1922–1923
Spaeth, Ralph	1931–1932
Stadler, Harold	1939–1941
Steward, Donald	1982–1985
Stintat-Ulich, Gisela	1954–1956
Stivrins, Patricia	1956–1959
Stryker, Winfield	1950–1951
Sturdevant, Raymond	1973–1976
Sujanski, Eva	1969–1971
Swanson, Jack	1971–1973
Sweeney, Michael	1978–1979
Swisher, William	1979–1982
Synhorst, David	1970–1971
Thomas, Julianne	1971–1974
Thomas, Patricia	1954–1955
Thorsteinsson, Geir	1961–1963
Trites, Barbara	1983–1986
Tweito, David	1966–1968
Ulich, Konrad	1954–1956
Ulich, Waltraud	1954–1956
Vazquez, Delia	1984–1985
Veenstra, Sallie	1978–1981
Verploeg, Ralph	1926–1927
Vinson, Robert	1958–1960
Visser, Valya	1973–1976
Von Behrn, Patricia	1970–1973
Von Hippel, Marianne	1963–1965
Votteler, Robert	1950–1951
Wagner, G. W.	1937–1939
Wallace, Peter	1969–1971
Walter, Andrew	1978–1981
Watts, A. F.	1917–1918
Welton, Michael	1970–1971
Weinstein, Mary	1972–1975
Weismann, Douglas	1973–1975
Weiss, Catherine	1982–1985
Whitworth, Rex	1949–1951
Wintermeyer, Keith	1982–1985
Wintermeyer, Laverne	1967–1968
Wispe, Jonathan	1979–1982
Wyatt, Richard	1974–1976
Yao, Chin C.	1968–1969
Younoszai, M. Kabir	1963–1964

Zarzour, Andre	1965–1966	Ziska, James	1967–1969
Zeaske, Richard	1968–1971		1971–1972
Zivkovich, Veljko	1969–1970		

Several other physicians have completed pediatric internships or portions of their pediatric training at the University of Iowa.

APPENDIX B

Postgraduate Fellowships in Pediatrics
University of Iowa Hospitals and Clinics

Name	*Fellowship*	*Dates*
Adedoyin, Michael	Gastroenterology	July 1975–June 1976
Ahrens, Richard	Allergy/Pulmonary	July 1977–July 1980
Andrews, Wayne	Neonatology/Nutrition	July 1976–July 1978
Arnett, Kenneth	Allergy/Pulmonary	July 1984–July 1986
Atkin, Joan	Genetics	July 1981–July 1983
Atkins, Dianne	Cardiology	July 1980–July 1983
Ayres, Nancy	Cardiology	July 1981–July 1984
Bapat, Vamana Rao	Hematology	July 1968–July 1969
Bayne, Edward	Cardiology	July 1977–July 1980
Bhatia, Jatinder	Neonatology/Nutrition	July 1979–July 1982
Binder, John	Developmental Disabilities	July 1976–July 1978
Birkbeck, John	Endocrinology	July 1960–July 1962
Bodensteiner, John	Neurology	July 1975–July 1976
Bosworth, Donna	Infectious Diseases	Sept 1979–Sept 1981
Brunberg, James	Neurology	July 1971–July 1973
Bryan, George	Endocrinology	July 1958–July 1959
Camacho, Jose	Cardiology	July 1984–July 1985
Carter, Guy	Cardiology	July 1973–July 1974
Cass, Kathleen	Cardiology	July 1980–July 1983
Chandramouli, B.	Cardiology	July 1967–July 1968
Cooke, Richard	Nutrition/Neonatology	July 1978–July 1980
Copeland, Linda	Developmental Disabilities	July 1984–July 1985
Danney, Mark	Endocrinology	July 1974–July 1976
Danso, Yunus	Ambulatory	July 1980–July 1981
Denison, Mark	Infectious Diseases	July 1983–July 1986
Dennis-Smithart, Ronda	Ambulatory	July 1985–July 1986
DeVizia, Basilio	Nutrition	July 1979–July 1980
Dunn, Amy	Ambulatory	July 1980–July 1981
Dusdieker, Lois	Ambulatory	July 1977–July 1979

Ehmke, Dorothy	Cardiology	July 1959–July 1962
Finch, Michael	Gastroenterology	July 1981–July 1983
Fleischaker, Gordon	Rheumatology	July 1958–July 1960
Florentine, Michael	Cardiology	July 1984–July 1985
Frank, Lee	Pharmacology	July 1974–July 1978
Garabedian, Hrair	Cardiology	July 1969–July 1971
Ghishan, Fayez	Gastroenterology	July 1977–July 1979
Gomez, Roberto	Nephrology	July 1980–July 1983
Gonzalez, Jose	Endocrinology	July 1980–July 1982
Grandgeorge, Steven	Allergy/Pulmonary	July 1984–Aug 1986
Green, Michael	Allergy/Pulmonary	July 1979–July 1981
Gyves, Peter	Endocrinology	July 1982–Dec 1984
Haddad, Nadra	Nutrition	July 1965–July 1966
Halmi, Katherine	Child Development	July 1968–July 1969
Harris, James	Allergy/Pulmonary	July 1983–July 1986
Haschke, Ferdinand	Nutrition	July 1979–July 1980
Hashimoto, Roopa	Ambulatory	July 1983–July 1986
Hayford, John	Endocrinology	July 1975–July 1977
Heck, Louis	Neonatology	July 1981–July 1983
Hendrix, James	Endocrinology	July 1977–July 1979
Hesz, Nancy	Developmental Disabilities	July 1983–July 1985
Humphries, C. Thomas	Allergy/Pulmonary	July 1983–July 1985
Husayni, Tarek	Cardiology	July 1981–July 1984
HuYoung, Alfred	Cardiology	July 1981–July 1983
Janco, Robert	Hematology/Oncology	July 1978–July 1981
Joad, Jesse	Allergy/Pulmonary	July 1982–July 1986
Karlsson, Maud	Ambulatory	July 1978–July 1980
Knight, Matthew	Ambulatory/Clin. Pharm.	July 1982–July 1985
Lababidi, Zuhdi	Cardiology	July 1968–July 1970
Larew, Mary	Infectious Diseases	July 1979–July 1981
Lee, Julia	Cardiology	July 1973–July 1978
Lyman, Margaret	Pulmonary/Cystic Fibrosis	July 1953–July 1956
MacMillan, Duncan	Endocrinology	July 1962–July 1964
Magurie, Grace	Infectious Diseases	July 1977–July 1979
Mahoney, Larry	Cardiology	July 1976–July 1979
Marvin, William	Cardiology	July 1975–July 1977
Matson, James	Nephrology	July 1977–July 1980
McDonnell, Jean	Child Development	July 1969–July 1970
McGuinness, Gail	Neonatology	July 1976–July 1977
McNeal, Douglas	Developmental Disabilities	July 1979–July 1981
Merrick, James	Allergy/Pulmonary	July 1981–July 1983
Mirhij, Najwa	Infectious Diseases	July 1976–May 1977

Mischler, Elaine	Cystic Fibrosis	July 1975–July 1977
Murph, Jody	Ambulatory	July 1982–July 1985
Najjar, Samir	Endocrinology	July 1959–July 1960
Nakamura, Kenneth	Neonatology	July 1982–July 1985
Nassif, Edward	Allergy/Pulmonary	July 1978–July 1980
Nathan, Radha	Gastroenterology	July 1978–July 1981
Nelsen, Carl	Nutrition/Metabolism	July 1963–July 1965
Normanly, Jerrod	Neurology	Jan. 1968–Dec. 1968
O'Donnell, Alejandro	Nutrition/Metabolism	July 1973–July 1974
Ovacik, Ekrem	Endocrinology	July 1962–July 1964
Overholt, Edward	Cardiology	July 1982–July 1985
Robillard, Jean	Nephrology	July 1973–July 1974
Sanchez, Lagrimas	Hematology/Oncology	July 1960–July 1962
Saunders, John	Neurology	July 1964–July 1966
Schultz, Frederick	Developmental Disabilities	July 1978–July 1980
Sell, Matthew	Neonatology	July 1983–July 1985
Shaw, Lein	Cardiology	July 1970–July 1971
Shaw, Robert	Neonatology	July 1978–July 1980
Sinning, Robert	Endocrinology	July 1960–July 1961
Sinno, Anwar	Neurology	July 1965–July 1967
Spiegel, Ronald	Neurology	July 1977–July 1980
Stillerman, Allan	Allergy/Pulmonary	July 1980–July 1983
Sweeney, Michael	Cardiology	July 1979–July 1980
Synhorst, David	Cardiology/Pharmacology	July 1971–July 1975
Thomas, Patricia	Rheumatology	July 1957–July 1958
Thorsteinsson, Geir	Genetics	July 1963–July 1964
Trembath, Jack	Developmental Disabilities	July 1961–July 1963
Tu, Jun-bi	Genetics	July 1964–July 1965
Vazquez, Delia	Endocrinology	July 1985–July 1986
Vazquez, Hector	Nutrition	July 1975–July 1976
VonBehrn, Patricia	Cardiology	July 1974–July 1977
Wagman, Armin	Cardiology	July 1983–July 1986
Waly, Farid	Cardiology	July 1971–July 1972
Weesner, Kenneth	Clinical Pharmacology	July 1981–July 1982
Weinstein, Mary	Neonatology	July 1975–July 1977
Weismann, Douglas	Nephrology/Pharmacology	July 1975–July 1977
Wispe, Jonathan	Neonatology/Pharmacology	July 1982–July 1985
Wolf, Stephen	Allergy/Pulmonary	July 1982–July 1984
Woodhead, Jerold	Nutrition/ Metab/Nephrology	July 1976–July 1979
Wyatt, Richard	Allergy/Pulmonary	July 1976–July 1978

Zataar, Rabih	Gastroenterology	July 1983–July 1986
Zivkovich, Veljko	Allergy/Pulmonary	July 1973–July 1977

Every attempt has been made to be as complete and accurate as possible. Any omission or error is unintentional.

APPENDIX C

Winners of the James C. Taylor Teaching Award in Pediatrics

1977 William E. Bell

1978 Martin G. Meyers

1978 Fred G. Smith, Jr.

1980 Jack Spevak

1981 Gail A. McGuinness

1982 Robert J. Roberts

1983 John T. Hayford

1984 Edward B. Clark

1985 Richard D. Andersen

1986 Pedro deAlarcon

APPENDIX D

Postgraduate Training Programs in Pediatrics at the University of Iowa Some Historical Perspectives

1870 State University College of Medicine opened, with a faculty of eight professors: 1) Surgery, 2) Theory and Practice of Medicine, 3) Materia Medica, 4) Physiology and Microscopical Anatomy, 5) Anatomy, 6) Obstetrics and Diseases of Women and Children, Dr. John Shrader, Chairman, 7) Chemistry and 8) Medical Jurisprudence.

1873 Mercy Hospital established in Iowa City, first hospital, had 87 general beds.

1892 Chair of Pathology and Bacteriology established with Walter Bierring as first Chairman.

1894 Dr. Bierring successfully produced diphtheria antitoxin. First produced in U.S. outside of New York.

1898 University Hospital (now Seashore Hall) completed and occupied (120 beds). Large wings added in 1907, 1913 and 1914 for total capacity of 350 beds. First hospital in Iowa with staff restricted to medical school faculty members.

1900 Bacteriology became a regular required course for all medical students.

1901 Medical building destroyed by fire.

1906 Dr. Charles S. Grant appointed as Instructor in Pediatrics in the Department of Theory and Practice of Medicine. Held position until 1915.

1909 Abraham Flexner's appraisal of U. of I. College of Medicine, visited in April, 1909: Iowa City's population in 9,007. "The clinical teachers are practitioners, some of them non-resident; the professor of Surgery resides in Sioux City; the professor of Gynecology, who is likewise Dean, at Dubuque."

1913 Dr. Arthur Steindler added to Iowa faculty in Orthopedics (but orthopedics not given separate departmental status until 1923).

1915 "Perkins Law" passed by Iowa Legislature, providing that "crippled children" could receive care at University Hospitals at State expense.

1915 Pediatrics established as a separate department in College of Medicine. Dr. Albert Byfield is chosen as first Department Head.

1917 Isolation Hospital for contagious diseases completed.

1918 Iowa Board of Medical Examiners require 1 year of internship for state licensing.

1919 Children's Hospital (now Steindler Building) opened. Was first building on west campus.

1924 Dr. P.C. Jeans chosen as Department Head in Pediatrics.

1925 New addition to Children's Hospital increases capacity to 240 beds (Rockefeller Foundation grant).

1927 Medical Laboratories building (basic sciences) completed on west campus.

1928 University Hospital completed on west campus.

1932 Hospital car services established.

1934 State Services for Crippled Children (SSCC) clinics (now CHSC) began as Orthopedic clinics under Dr. Steindler.

1936 Iowa SSCC formally organized to include Pediatrics and Orthopedics.

1952 Dr. Charles May becomes Department Head in Pediatrics.

1954 Pediatrics moved from Children's Hospital to 1-West of University Hospitals.

1954 Hospital School for Severely Handicapped Children completed.

1957 Medical Research Center completed (Connecting Medical Labs to University Hospital).

1958 Dr. Wallace McCrory chosen Department Head in Pediatrics.

1960 First Pediatric Surgeon at Iowa, Dr. R. T. Soper, joins the Department of Surgery.

1960 Chromosome Lab opened.

1961 Dr. Donal Dunphy becomes Department Head in Pediatrics.

1964 South Wing added to Hospital School.

1966 Straight pediatric internship introduced.

1967 Adolescent ward opens on 5-South.

1968 Neonatal Transport Van begins operation under direction of Dr. George Baker. The first vehicle is a converted bread truck.

1968 Infant ICU opens 1W-104, 4 beds.

1970 2 West Pediatrics (Adolescent) and Pediatric Surgical Ward opens (Remodeled 1971–72 and ward moved temporarily to C-51).

1973 Dr. Fred Smith chosen Department Head in Pediatrics.

1975 First NICU opened on 4-West, 12 beds.

1978 High Risk Infant Follow-up Program started.

1979 Aircare became operational.

1981 4-West Intermediate Nursery opened, PICU opened.

1982 Limited phlebotomy service instituted in Pediatrics.

1982 New 11-bed NICU opened, Newborn Nursery remodeled.

1982 Pediatric Clinic, Adolescent ward, Infant and Toddler wards and Intermediate Intensive Care Unit opened in John Colloton Pavilion.

1985 Ronald McDonald House opened.

1986 Pediatric Bone Marrow Transplant Unit opens on 7RCE.

1987 Frank Morriss, Jr., becomes Professor and Head of Pediatrics.

APPENDIX E

Selected Medical Milestones of Relevance to Pediatrics
(After Fielding Garrison)

460–370 B.C.	Hippocrates. Refers to special features of diseases as they occur in children, ie. his treatise, "on dentition."
98–117 A.D.	Soranus of Ephesus writings *On disease of women* contain a treatise on children's diseases: first medical reference to rickets.
131–201	Galen, founder of experimental physiology. Refers to children's diseases incidentally throughout his writings.
860–932	Rhazes, first accurate accounts of smallpox and measles. The first physician to write an entire treatise on diseases of children.
1100s	Anonymous 12th-century manuscript *The children's practice* is written. It provides common sense advice in child care, probably compiled from the work of earlier Greek and Arabian writers. Appears in different formats for 400 years.
1137	St. Bartholomew's Hospital founded (London).
1444	Spedale degli Innocenti (Hospital of the Little Foundlings) opens in Florence, Italy.
1452–1519	Leonardo da Vinci.
1472	Bagellardo's *Libellus de Egritidinibus Infantium* published in Padua: first printed book dealing exclusively with pediatrics.
1493–1551	Paracelsus.
1500	Nufer performs first successful caesarian section on living subject (his wife).
1513	Rosslin's *Rosengarten* published in Strassburg containing chapters on feeding and care of infants and diseases of children; more than 100 editions in over 200 years.
1514–64	Vesalius. *Fabrica* published 1543, forms foundation of modern anatomy.

1530 Fracastorius, physician-poet, publishes medical poem *Syphilis sive Morbus Gallius,* describing contemporary dietetic and therapeutic knowledge, recognizing venereal cause and gives the disease its name (Venice).
1546 Phayre's *Regiment of Life* published containing first English pediatric writings (*The Boke of Children*).
1553 Servetus describes the pulmonary circulation.
1565 Nicot brings tobacco plant to France.
1575 Baillon describes laryngeal croup as a new disease.
1578 Baillon first describes whooping cough.
1581 Rousset publishes treatise on Caesarian section.
1584 Sir Walter Raleigh brings curare from Guiana to England.
1590 Hans and Zacharias Janssen invent compound microscope.
1628 Harvey's *De Motu Cordis* published, Frankfurt.
1639 First printing press in North America (Cambridge, Mass.)
1650 Glisson describes rickets in *De rachitide.*
1653 Robert Pemell's *Treatise of the diseases of children* published (London). Second pediatric text written in English.
1656 First intravenous injection of drugs performed by Sir Christopher Wren, Boyle and Wilkens in dogs.
1661 Malpighi gives first description of capillary system.
1661 De Graaf shows that ova develop in the ovary.
1664 Willis's *Cerebri anatome* is published.
1667 Willis book on pathology of the brain published; contains reference to convulsions in children.
1670 Willis describes sweet taste of diabetic urine.
1670 Thomas Sydenham publishes an accurate description of measles.
1673 Leeuwenhoek makes microscopes.
1675 Sydenham publishes first description of scarlet fever.
1689 Walter Harris (a protege of Syndenham) publishes *De morbis acute infantum* (London). Proposes use of alkalis in the treatment of infants as "all the complaints of infants spring from an acid as their common source."
1697 John Pechey publishes *General Treatise of the Disease of Infants,* London.
1714 Fahrenheit constructs 212° thermometer.
1717 Blair gives earliest description of pyloric stenosis.
1740 Hoffman describes rubella.
1741 Andry's *Orthopedia* published; first work devoted to orthopedic problems in children.
1742 Celsius invents 100-degree thermometer.
1748 William Cadogan publishes *An essay upon nursing, and the management of children, from their birth to three years of age* (London).

1765	Rosen von Rosenstein's book *The diseases of children and their remedies* published (Stockholm). Notable for its scientific outlook.
1767	Herberden describes varicella.
1768	Robert Whytt of Edinburgh provides first accurate description of tuberculous meningitis.
1771	Armstrong describes congenital pyloric stenosis.
1771–74	Priestly and Schule isolate oxygen.
1777	Lavoisier describes process of gas exchange occuring in lungs with respiration.
1783	Mellin publishes book on diseases of children.
1784	Michael Underwood's *Treatise on the diseases of children* published (London). Contains first description of sclerema neonatorum (Underwood's disease) and infantile poliomyelitis and also gives accurate description of thrush and rickets.
1784	Cotugno discovers cerebrospinal fluid.
1785	Withering's book on digitalis published.
1796	Jenner performs first innoculation, publishes results in 1798 in An *Inquiry into the Causes and Effects of the Variolae Vaccinae.*
1803	Otto describes hemophilia.
1806	Vieusseux describes first outbreak of "cerebrospinal" (meningococcal) meningitis in Geneva, Switzerland.
1816	Laennec invents stethoscope.
1822–84	Gregor Mendel.
1826	Bretonneau describes diphtheritis.
1826	Dupuytren describes congenital dislocation of the hip.
1835	C. P. Louis founds medical statistics.
1837	Flourens describes respiratory center in medulla.
1839	Diffenbach operates successfully for strabismus.
1840	West in London writes letter to editor of *Lancet* describing his son's "massive spasms," later referred to as infantile spasm or West's Syndrome.
1840	Heine describes infantile paralysis.
1843	First pediatric journal published in Berlin, *Journal Fuer Kinderkrankheiten.*
1846	Hutchison invents spirometer.
1846	Virchow and Hughes Bennett describe leukemia.
1846–47	Ether and Chloroform anesthesia, introduced by Morton, Bigelow, Simpson and others.
1846	Bernard describes digestive function of pancreas.
1846	American Medical Association founded.
1847	Semmelweis describes pathogenesis of puerperal fever.
1848	Fehling introduces test for glucosuria.

1849	Sedillot performs gastrostomy.
1850	Gavage feeding of small infants described by Marchant at meeting of Academy of Medicine.
1851	Helmholz invents opthalmoscope.
1852	Hospital for Sick Children in Great Ormond Street opens, London, England.
1855	Garcia introduces laryngoscope.
1855	Children's Hospital of Philadelphia opens (First permanent Pediatric hospital in America).
1855	Addison describes adrenal insufficiency.
1857	Denuce describes use of incubator to warm the premature infant. (First published report of incubator use in the premature infant).
1857	Borden operates first station for sanitary inspection of milk in New York.
1858	Diday, in Paris, writes classic monograph on syphilis in the newborn.
1859	Lacock, an obstetrician (to the Queen of England) finds bromides to be useful to control central "attacks"—later seizures.
1860	Schultze introduces a method of resuscitating asphyxiated neonates.
1860	Jacobi opens first American pediatric clinic, N.Y. Medical College.
1867	Lister introduces antiseptic surgery.
1868	Duchenne, a French neurologist, describes "pseudohypertrophic muscular paralysis"—later called muscular dystrophy.
1871	Hutchison performs first successful operation on child with intussusception.
1872	American Public Health Association holds first meeting.
1874	Henoch describes purpura in children.
1875	Barlow describes scurvy in infants.
1875	Society for the Prevention of Cruelty to Children established.
1876–77	Germ theory of infectious diseases advanced by Pasteur and Koch.
1879	Neisser discovers gonnococcus.
1880	Pasteur discovers streptococcus, staphylococcus and pneumococcus.
1880	Section on Pediatrics of AMA established by Jacobi.
1881	Medin describes epidemic nature of poliomyelitis.
1882	O'Dwyer reports successful treatment of diphtheric croup by intubation.
1882	Koch discovers tubercle bacillus is cause of "consumption."

1883 Klebs discovers diphtheria bacillus.

1884 Neonatal opthalmoprophylaxis introduced by Crede using silver nitrate.

1884 *Archives of Pediatrics* begins publication. First paper titled "Convulsions in Childhood" by W. T. Plant of Syracuse.

1885 A. Meigs publishes analysis of human milk in *Milk Analysis and Infant Feeding.*

1886 Down publishes paper on "mongolism" which he attributes to tuberculosis in the parents.

1886 Venle in England names a measles-like exanthem, rubella.

1886 Escherich describes intestinal bacterial flora of infants.

1886–87 Hirschsprung describes features of megacolon and pyloric stenosis.

1887 Weichalbaum first describes Neisseria meningititis in purulent CSF.

1887 Babies Hospital founded in New York City, the first American hospital devoted exclusively to care of infants and children.

1888 Roux and Yersin isolate diphtheria toxin.

1888 Section on Pediatrics split off from section on Internal Medicine of AMA for separate presentation of papers.

1888 American Pediatric Society founded by 43 pediatricians, Jacobi first president.

1888 Fallot describes tetralogy of cardiac defects associated with his name.

1889 Conn investigates bacteriology of milk.

1890 Pasteurization of milk begun on a commercial scale in Denmark.

1890 Behring and Kitasato prepare diphtheria antitoxin.

1891 Quincke introduces lumbar puncture.

1891 Halsted introduces rubber gloves in operative surgery.

1891 Hedin invents hematocrit.

1892 Certified milk introduced by Coit in New Jersey.

1892 Pfeiffer first identifies haemophilus influenzae, later called "Pfeiffer's bacillus," erroneously believed to be the cause of the influenza pandemic of 1891–1892.

1892 Osler's *The Principles and Practice of Medicine* published.

1894 Townsend introduces term "haemorrhagic disease of the newborn" to describe a form of generalized bleeding occurring in newborns.

1894 Dukes describes "Fourth disease."

1895 First American newborn nursery established at Johns Hopkins Hospital.

1895 Roentgen discovers X-rays.

1896 Arthritis deformans described by Still (Still's disease).

1897 First X-ray department for infants and children opens, Graz, Austria.
1897 Holt's *The Diseases of Infancy and Childhood* published.
1898 Rubner and Heubner publish monograph on metabolism and average caloric needs of the normal and "atrophic" infant. Formed basis for modern investigations on infant metabolism.
1898 Marfan describes use of superior sagittal sinus for administration of intravenous fluids and blood drawing.
1898 Ferguson of Chicago attempts first surgical shunting for hydrocephalus using shunt from lumbar subarachnoid space to peritoneum.
1898 Babinski, student of Charcot, publishes the significance of great toe extension with plantar stimulation, later called the Babinski sign.
1898 Martin Couney (associate of P. Budin) exhibits premature infants in Tarnier incubators at the World Exposition in Berlin.
1899 Acetylsalicylic acid introduced.
1900 Park recommends control of milk bacterial tests (New York City).
1900 Pierre Budin publishes *Le Nourisson* outlining basic principles of care for premature infants (Paris).
1901 Landsteiner discovers blood types (iso-aglutination) A, B, O.
1902 McClung isolates sex chromosome.
1905 Hirschsprung describes use of hydrostatic pressure to reduce intussusception.
1905 Bordatella pertussis cultured by Bordet and Gengou.
1905 Schaudinn and Hoffmann show the cause of syphilis is a spirochaete (Berlin).
1906 Winter resuscitates heart using adrenalin injections.
1906 Landsteiner introduces the dark-field microscope to detect *spirochaetes* (syphilis).
1906 Flexner introduces antimeningococcal horse serum—the first specific drug therapy for meningitis, reduces mortality to 30%.
1906 Von Pirquet coins term "allergy" to denote altered tissue reactivity.
1906 National Committee on Child Labor established (USA).
1906 Wasserman introduces serum diagnosis of syphilis.
1907 First large epidemic of poliomyelitis reported in New York.
1908 Darling first reports patients with histoplasmosis.
1908 Chicago adopts compulsory pasteurization of milk.

1908 Van Reuss first describes galactosemia.
1908 Garrod introduces concept of inborn errors of metabolism, first applying it to alkaptonuria, albinism, cystinuria and pentosuria.
1908–09 Antenatal hygiene started in New York and Boston.
1909 First White House conference on Children and Youth.
1910 Adrenogenital syndrome recognized by Apert.
1910 Ehrlich and Hata introduce salvarsan.
1910 Zahorsky describes roseola infantum.
1910 American Association for Study and Prevention of Infant Mortality formed.
1911 *American Journal of Diseases of Children* begins publication.
1912 Hauptmann in Germany introduces phenobarbital for treatment of seizures.
1912 Ramstedt operation for pyloric stenosis developed.
1912 First full-time pediatric clinic in the U.S. opens at Johns Hopkins Hospital.
1912 Children's Bureau of U.S. Department of Labor founded.
1912 Wilson describes hepatolenticular degeneration.
1913 X-ray diagnosis of intussusception made by Ladd.
1913 Active immunization for diphtheria first introduced, improved in 1923.
1914 Holt, Courtney and Fales describe chemical composition of diarrheal stools.
1915 Howland and Marriott prove that infants with severe diarrhea are in a state of acidosis, recommend administration of sodium bicarbonate.
1917 von Wagner-Jauregg introduces malarial therapy for treatment of tertiary syphilis, awarded Nobel prize for his work in 1927.
1917 Schloss recommends intravenous route for administration of fluids in pediatric patients.
1917 Bloch describes Xeropthalmia in children (Vitamin A Deficiency).
1917–19 Work of Van Slyke and Folin allows measurement of serum chemistries.
1918 Dandy describes pneumoencephalography.
1918 Waterhouse-Friderichsen syndrome described.
1919 Marriott recognizes importance of volume depletion in severe diarrhea, recommends intraperitoneal fluid replacement.
1919 Huldschinsky demonstrates curative effect of sunlight on rickets.

1920 National Child Health Council organized (USA).
1921 Sheppard-Towner Act signed into law (Indirectly led to founding of American Academy of Pediatrics).
1921 Abt introduces first electric breast pump.
1921 Howland and Kramer describe calcium x phosphorus product and its relationship to the severity of rickets.
1922 Insulin discovered by Banting. Its use in children was described in 1923 by Cowie and Parsons.
1923 Dick and Dick discover hemolytic streptococcus of scarletina.
1923 Murlin identifies glucagon.
1923 Coca and Cooke introduce word atopy to describe an abnormal hypersensitivity distinct from serum sickness and anaphylaxis.
1924 Calmette vaccinates children against tuberculosis with B.C.G.
1924 First electroencephalogram recorded by Berger. First published in German in 1929, first recordings done on his son.
1925 Thalassemia described by Cooley.
1925 Hart reports first successful exchange transfusion in an infant with familial icterus gravis. Uses anterior fontanel and saphenous vein.
1925 McCollum names antirachitic factor in cod-liver oil Vitamin D.
1926 *Journal of Pediatrics* begins publication.
1926 Harington identifies thyroxine.
1927 Vitamin B1 (thiamin) named (antineuritic factor).
1927 Vitamin B2 (riboflavin) named (synthesized in 1935).
1927 Smith describes thyroid stimulating hormone.
1928 Vitamin C isolated by Szent-Gyorgy.
1928 Penicillin discovered by Fleming.
1929 Society for Pediatric Research founded.
1929 Gamble, Butler and McKhann report loss of intracellular potassium during diarrhea.
1930 Coburn implicates Group A hemolytic streptococci as cause of tissue reactions in rheumatic fever.
1930 American Academy of Pediatrics organized.
1930 Vitamin D isolated by Bourdillon.
1931 Fanconi describes child with rickets, stunted growth, albuminuria and glycosuria (Fanconi Syndrome).
1932 Bilateral adrenal hyperplasia described by Cushing.
1932 Blackfan, Diamond and Baty use term erythroblastosis fetalis to describe clinical syndromes of icterus gravis neonatorum, congenital anemia of the newborn and hydrops fetalis.

1933 Lancefield at Rockefeller Institute first classified streptocci on basis of cell wall carbohydrate composition.
1933 Rich and McCordock from Johns Hopkins describe pathogenesis of tuberculous meningitis.
1933 Ladd describes intestinal malrotation and its surgical treatment.
1933 American Board of Pediatrics established.
1933 Electrophoresis introduced by Tiselius.
1933 Sauer reports results of pertussis vaccine trials in *JAMA*.
1934 Folling describes phenylketonuria.
1934 Dam discovers Vitamin K.
1935 Federal Social Security Act introduced.
1935 Antibiotic era begins with sulfachrysoidine (Protnosil), introduced by Domagk. First used in U. S. at Columbia University in New York for treatment of a 10-year-old girl with Hemophilus influenzae meningitis.
1935 Fanconi, Uehlinger and Knauer publish first paper on cystic fibrosis.
1936 Cortisone (Compound E) isolated by Mason, Meyers and Kendall.
1936 Vitamin E isolated by Evans and Emerson.
1936 Evans and colleagues describe FSH, LH.
1937 Nicotinic acid isolated by Subbarow.
1937 Seibert develops purified protein derivative (PPD).
1938 Surgical closure of patent ductus arteriosus performed by Gross.
1938 First diagnostic use of I^{131} in children by Reilly and associates.
1938 Deoxycorticosterone isolated by Reichstein.
1938 Blackfan and Diamond describe hypoplastic anemia.
1938 Trask and colleagues isolate poliomyelitis virus from stools of patient with abortive poliomyelitis.
1938 Putnam and Merritt introduce Dilantin (diphenylhydantoin sodium) for epilepsy.
1938 Fry in London first reports fatal cases of puerperal sepsis caused by Group B streptococcus.
1939 First American Professorship in Pediatric surgery established by Harvard.
1939 Wolf and colleagues describe congenital toxoplasma infection.
1939 Ladd and Leven develop multiple stage treatment of tracheo-esophageal atresia.
1941 Landsteiner and Weiner discover Rh factor.
1941 First patient treated with penicillin, Oxford, England. Reported by Abraham, Chain and associates in *Lancet*.

1941 Martin and Synge introduce chromatography for analysis of protein hydrolysates.
1941 Levine and associates show that the Rh factor is related to the pathogenesis of erythroblastosis fetalis.
1941 Gregg observes congenital defects in offspring of mothers with rubella in pregnancy in Australia.
1942 Terry describes retrolental fibroplasia, association with oxygen reported by Campbell in 1951.
1943 Mahoney first publishes use of penicillin for treatment of syphilis at Public Health Hospital on Staten Island, N.Y.
1944 Helfrick and Abelson describe use of total parenteral nutrition in an infant with Hirschsprung's disease.
1944 Streptomycin discovered by Schatz, Bogie and Waksman.
1944 Cohn and colleagues introduce use of human immune serum globulin (gamma globulin) in passive prophylaxis of measles.
1944 Weiner and Wexler report exchange transfusion for erythroblastosis fetalis using radial artery and saphenous vein.
1945 Blalock and Taussig describe shunting technique which bears their name.
1945 Crafoord and Nylin and Gross independently treat coarctation of the aorta surgically.
1946 Diamond and coworkers introduce technique of umbilical vein catheterization for exchange transfusion.
1946 Paraaminosalicylic acid (PAS) introduced.
1946 Spock's book *Baby and Child Care* first published.
1946 Barr and Bertram describe sex chromatin.
1946 Darrow describes the importance of potassium replacement in infants with severe diarrhea.
1946 di Sant'Agnese and Andersen report use of antibiotics to treat lung disease in cystic fibrosis.
1947 Dalldorf and Sickles describe Coxsackie viruses.
1947 Chloramphenicol isolated.
1947 Exchange transfusion for erythroblastosis fetalis performed by Diamond using umbilical vein.
1948 Chlortetracycline isolated by Duggar.
1948 Rickes isolates Vitamin B_{12}.
1948 Farber describes use of aminopterin to induce remission in ALL.
1948 *Pediatrics* begins publication.
1949 Pauling and associates clarify the molecular structure of hemoglobin S, initiating the era of molecular biology.
1949 Neomycin isolated.
1949 Nelson and Mayer introduce the first treponemal test—the TPI.

1950 Dicke describes gluten-free diet to treat celiac disease.
1950 Hemoglobin C described by Itano and Neel.
1950 Wilkins describes suppression of androgen secretion with cortisone.
1950 Duffy and Fitzgerald describe association between radiation therapy in infancy and thyroid sarcoma.
1950 Dean reports on mass fluoridation of water to prevent dental caries.
1950 National Science Foundation established.
1951 Isoniazid (INH) introduced; *New York Times* has front page photo of patients literally "dancing in the streets."
1951 Gallager organizes first adolescents' unit in U.S. in Boston.
1952 Tetracycline produced.
1952 Apgar proposes method of evaluation of newborn that bears her name.
1952 AAP establishes an Accident Prevention Committee.
1952 Bruton describes agammaglobulinemia.
1952 Erythromycin introduced by McGuire.
1952 Brock and Autret describe protein calorie malnutrition (Kwashiorkor).
1952 Nulson and Spitz in Philadelphia introduce the Holter valve enabling vascular shunts from the ventricles.
1953 Watson and Crick describe DNA double helix.
1953 Hyaline Membrane Disease described as a pathological entity in premature infants.
1953 First successful correction of an intracardiac defect (atrial septal defect) with cardiopulmonary bypass.
1953 Hypothermia used in surgical treatment of ASD by Lewis.
1953 Aldosterone tested.
1953 Oxytocin synthesized by duVigneaud.
1953 di Sant'Agnese and colleagues describe swest electrolyte abnormalities in cystic fibrosis. Basis for diagnostic sweat test.
1954 Menkes and others describe maple syrup urine disease.
1954 Salk vaccine (inactivated poliovirus vaccine) introduced.
1954 Ramos-Alvarez and Sabin describe ECHO virus infections.
1954 Aldrich of Mayo Clinic Department of Pediatrics describes (in *Pediatrics*) a north-central Iowa family with x-linked disorder characterized by eczema, recurrent infections and thrombocytopenia—later called Wiscott-Aldrich syndrome.
1955 Amphotericin B isolated.
1955 Lillehei and colleagues report first complete intracardiac repair of tetralogy of Fallot.
1955 Salk introduces inactivated polio vaccine.
1956 Carson describes congenital hemolytic anemia caused by G-6-PD deficiency.

1957 Kanamycin isolated by Umezawa.
1958 Phototherapy for prevention of hyperbilirubinemia introduced.
1959 Avery and Mead demonstrate that lungs of infants dying from hyaline membrane disease are surfactant-deficient.
1959 Chromosomal defect of Down's syndrome described by Lejeune.
1959 Ford reports chromosome abnormalities in Klinefelter's syndrome and Turner's syndrome.
1959 Pilocarpine iontophoresis for diagnosis of cystic fibrosis described by Gibson and Cooke.
1960 Newell and Hungerford report Philadelphia chromosome in patients with chronic myelogenous leukemia.
1960 Methicillin, first semisynthetic, penicillinase resistant penicillin introduced.
1960 ACTH synthesized by Hofmann.
1961 Kempe coins term "battered child syndrome" calling attention to child abuse.
1961 National Institute of Child Health and Human Development founded.
1962 Taussig describes congenital malformations caused by thalidomide.
1962 Sabin introduces live, attenuated polio vaccine.
1963 Encephalopathy and fatty degeneration of the viscera (Reyes' Syndrome) described.
1963 Lubchenco et al. publish intrauterine growth percentile chart.
1963 Measles vaccine (live attenuated measle virus) licensed.
1963 RhoGAM introduced by Freda.
1964 Gell and Coombs classify allergic reactions into 4 types: Type I–Type IV.
1966 Rashkind balloon septostomy described.
1966 Steele and Breg report successful karyotyping of amniotic cells ushering in era of prenatal diagnosis.
1966 Ishizaka, Ishizaka and colleagues identify IgE as human reaginic antibody.
1967 Bronchopulmonary dysplasia first described by Northway and coworkers.
1967 Mucocutaneous lymph node syndrome described by Kawasaki.
1968 Henle, Henle and Diehl report association of infectious mononucleosis and Epstein-Barr virus.
1969 Rubella vaccine (live attenuated virus) licensed.
1969 Hounsfield develops computerized transverse axial scanning (CAT scan). First EMI scanner operational 1972.

1971 Continuous positive airway pressure described by Gregory and associates.
1971 AMA urges adoption of regionalized perinatal programs.
1973 First isolates recovered of ampicillin resistant Haemophilus influenza strains in U.S. in Maryland.
1976 Immotile cilia syndrome described by Afzelius, Pedersen and Mygrind.
1977 PL 94-142 implemented allowing "mainstreaming" of disabled children.
1977 Dubowitz and Dubowitz publish clinical manual "Gestational Age of the Newborn."
1980 Fujiwara and associates report the use of an artificial surfactant therapy in hyaline membrane disease.
1981 Acquired immune deficiency syndrome (AIDS) described.
1985 Localization of cystic fibrosis gene locus to chromosome 7.
1986 Localization of the gene defect in Duchenne muscular dystrophy on the X-chromosome by Louis Kunkel and colleagues.

APPENDIX F

Bibliography

Books

Abt AF and Garrison F. History of Pediatrics. Philadelphia: W. B. Saunders, 1965.

Baker SJ. Child hygiene. New York: Harper, 1923.

Bettman OL. The good old days—they were terrible! New York: Random House, 1974.

Bierring W. A History of the Department of Internal Medicine State University of Iowa College of Medicine 1870–1958. Iowa City: State University of Iowa, 1958.

Boyd WR. A brief history of the College of Medicine of the Iowa State University, 1909–1934, n.p., 1934, University of Iowa Archives.

Bradbury DE and Stoddard GD. Pioneering in Child Welfare Iowa Child Welfare Research Station 1917–1938. Iowa City: State University of Iowa, 1933.

Cone TE. History of American Pediatrics. Boston: Little, Brown and Company, 1979.

Cone CB. History of the State University of Iowa: The College of Medicine. 1934, The University of Iowa Archives.

Faber HK and MacIntosh R. History of the American Pediatric Society 1887–1965. New York: McGraw-Hill, 1966.

Flexner A. Medical Education in the United States and Canada. New York: Arno Press, Inc., 1972.

Garrison F. History of Medicine. Philadelphia: W.B. Saunders, 1929.

Iowa Medical Society. One Hundred Years of Iowa Medicine. Iowa City: Athens Press, 1950.

Keettel WC. A History of the Department of Obstetrics and Gynecology–The University of Iowa 1848–1980. Iowa City: The University of Iowa, 1981.

Means JH. The Associations of American Physicians, Its First Seventy-five Years. New York: McGraw-Hill, 1961.

Rothstein WG. American Physicians of the Nineteenth Century. Baltimore: Johns Hopkins Press, 1972.

Smith CA. The Children's Hospital of Boston "Built Better Than They Knew." Boston: Little, Brown and Co., 1983.

Shaw WB., ed. The University of Michigan: An Encyclopedic Survey. Ann Arbor: University of Michigan Press, 1951; Vol II, pp. 899–904.

Still GF. The history of pediatrics. Oxford: Oxford University Press, 1931.

25th Anniversary Report and 50th Anniversary Report, Harvard College Class of 1902. Cambridge: The University Press, 1927 and 1952.

Articles

Bean WB. America's first coeducational medical school. Journal of the Iowa Medical Society 1970; 60:237.

Blackfan KD. Past Presidents of the American Pediatric Society 1888–1938, President's Address. Am J Dis Child 1938; 56:1.

Buckwalter JA. Arthur Steindler: founder of Iowa Orthopedics. The Iowa Orthopedic Journal 1981; 1:5–12.

Cone TE. Highlights of two centuries of American pediatrics, 1776–1976. Am J Dis Child 1976; 130:771.

Cooke JV. How's your medical orthoëpy? Washington University Medical Alumni Quarterly 1943; 6:231.

Death Notice–P. C. Jeans. JAMA 1952; 150:1500.

Holt LE. Infant mortality ancient and modern. An historical sketch. Arch Pediatr 1913; 30:885.

Landsberger M. Some pediatric milestones of the 19th century. Am J Dis Child 1964; 108:206.

Pearson HA. Lectures on the diseases of children by Eli Ives, M.D. of Yale and New Haven: America's First Academic Pediatrician. Pediatrics 1986; 77:680–686.

Schweltzer CR. A developmental history of the State Services for Crippled Children's Program in Iowa. MA thesis, University of Iowa School of Social Work, 1951.

Silverman WA. Incubator–baby side shows. Pediatrics 1979; 64:127–141.

Smith RM. Medicine as a science: Pediatrics. N Engl J Med 1951; 244:176.

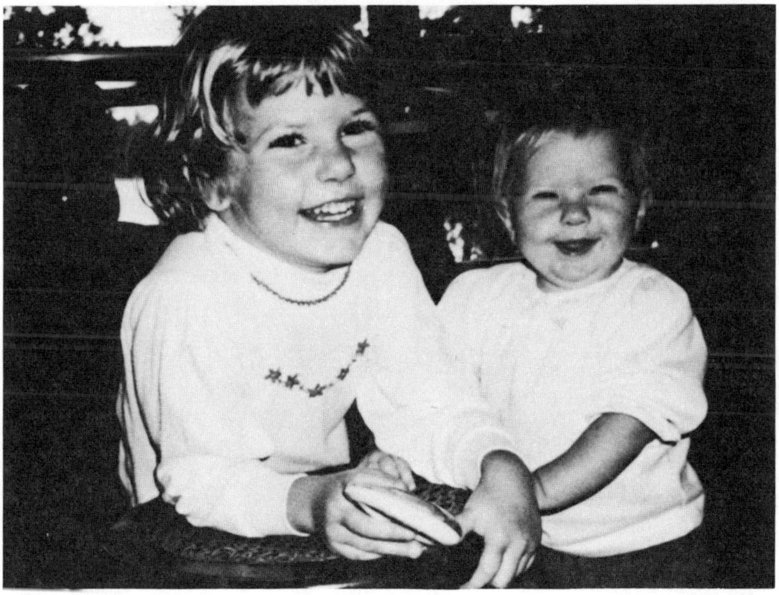

Maggie and Rebecca McCray
Ages 4 and 1 Years
July, 1986